PLANT BASED PCOS DIET COOKBOOK

Empower your health with 1000 days of Plant-Powered recipes for hormonal balance, PCOS management, fertility boost, and weight loss with the insulin resistance diet

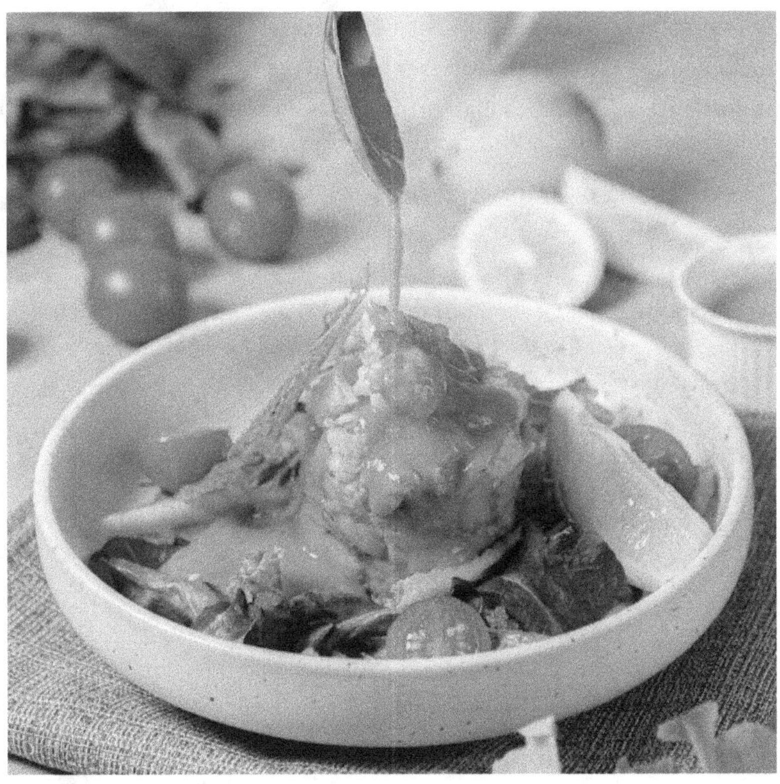

Caroline Maryse

If you have any questions, insights, or if there's anything specific you'd like to discuss regarding the content of this book, feel free to reach out. Your feedback is valuable, and I'm here to support you on your wellness journey.

You can email me at wellnesswithcarolinemaryse@gmail.com. I'll do my best to respond promptly and provide the assistance you may need. Your well-being is important, and I'm dedicated to ensuring your experience with this book is enriching and empowering.

TABLE OF CONTENT

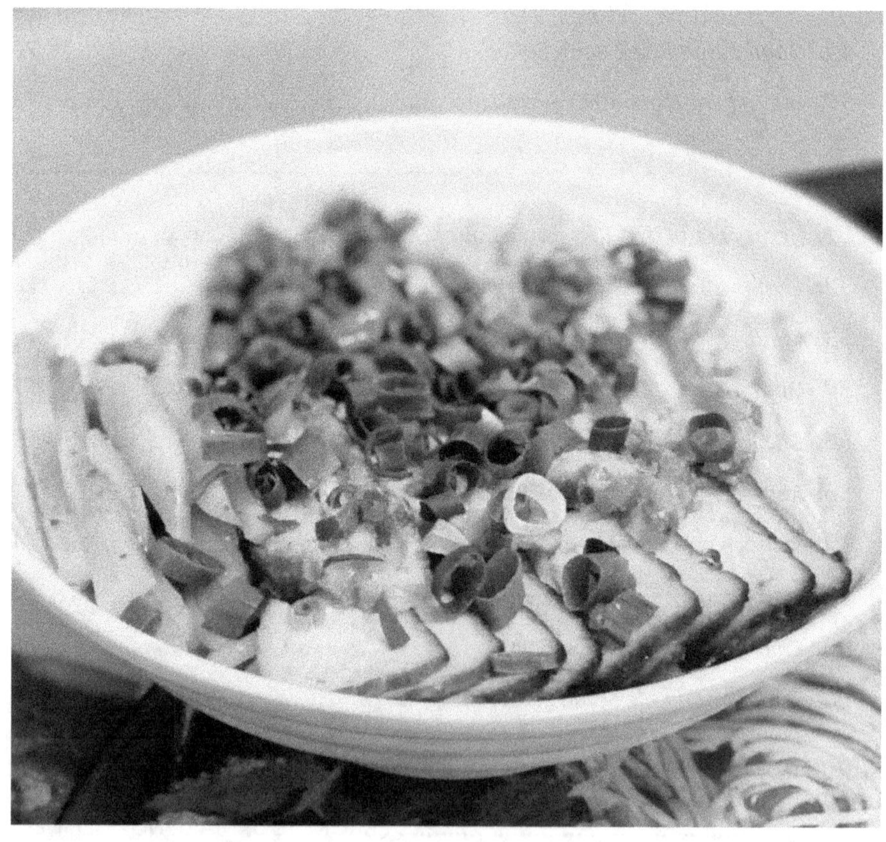

Have you ever felt that your body is trying to communicate with you but you don't comprehend what its saying? Have you struggled with hormone imbalances, PCOS management, reproductive issues, and the complicated dance of weight reduction and insulin resistance? You're not alone if you're nodding along, sensing a connection inside your own experience.

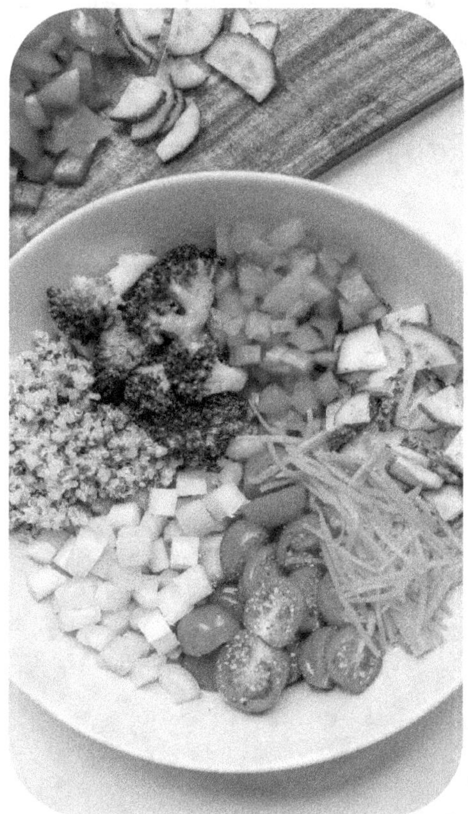

Consider a dynamic person navigating the maze of life, someone who, like you, has struggled with the difficulties of PCOS. This person began a serious examination, not just of the ailment, but also of the transforming power of plant-based life.

That person is me. The ups and downs, wins and defeats—it's a story that many of us can relate to. The Plant-Based PCOS Diet Cookbook gets its inspiration from this story.

In the pages that follow, I'll take you on a journey, not just through recipes, but also through my own voyage. An adventure that grew into a dedication to plant-powered living, a holistic approach to wellbeing that has transformed my relationship with food, health, and, eventually, my life.

This cookbook is a guide, a partner in your search for hormonal balance, PCOS treatment, fertility improvement, and weight loss with the insulin resistance diet. Each meal is a component of a greater puzzle, designed to nourish your body and spirit while also empowering your health in ways that go beyond the limits of traditional diets.

Discover the thrill of vivid, nutrient-rich meals tailored to your own path. Each meal, from morning delights to enticing sweets, is a celebration of flavor and well-being.

The advantages go beyond the plate—this is a lifestyle change that corresponds to your body's requirements, a sensitive approach to self-care that extends well beyond the kitchen.

It's as easy to navigate the cookbook as it is to enjoy a well-crafted dish. Dive into the chapters, each of which demonstrates a distinct aspect of your well-being. Begin by learning about PCOS and acquiring insights that will help you understand it better. Adopt a comprehensive approach to wellbeing by indulging in plant-based treats that feed your body at every turn.

As you begin on your culinary adventure, utilize the accompanying meal plans to guide your week and the shopping lists to make your trip to the grocery store easier. This cookbook is intended to be an ally, a source of inspiration, and a guide to a better, more balanced self. Allow the bright recipes, personal tales, and practical recommendations in the pages that follow to serve as your compass on this journey toward a plant-powered, PCOS-friendly lifestyle.

Welcome to a transforming journey that goes beyond the pages of a cookbook and becomes a vital chapter in your own wellness narrative.

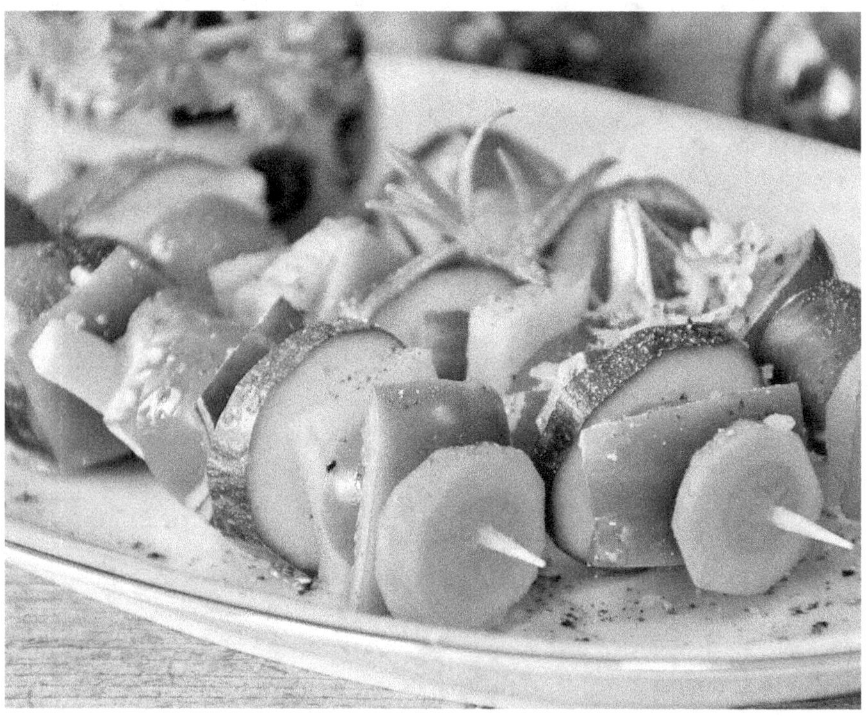

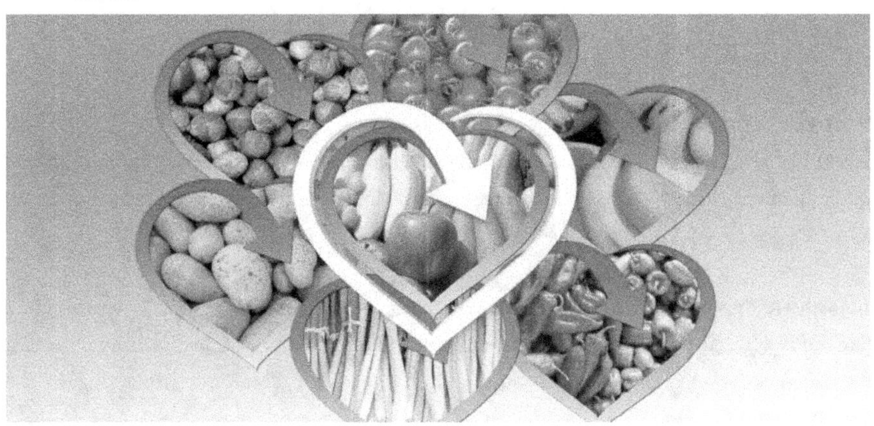

INTRODUCTION TO PCOS

Polycystic Ovary Syndrome, or PCOS, is a complicated and frequent health disorder that affects people, particularly women, in a variety of ways. As we begin our quest to comprehend PCOS, it is critical that we understand the essential features that identify and describe this illness.

PCOS is characterized by hormonal imbalances, ovarian cysts, and a variety of symptoms that can have a negative influence on a person's overall health. It is one of the most frequent endocrine diseases in women of reproductive age, with a geographically diverse frequency. While the precise origin of PCOS is unknown, it is largely accepted that it is impacted by a mix of genetic, environmental, and lifestyle factors.

The path to a PCOS diagnosis can be difficult for many people, generally highlighted by the discovery of symptoms such as irregular menstrual cycles, higher levels of androgens (male hormones), and the existence of polycystic ovaries. However, it is critical to understand that PCOS is a spectrum condition, which means that its symptoms can vary greatly across individuals.

Aside from its reproductive consequences, PCOS is rapidly becoming recognized for its link to a variety of metabolic and cardiovascular concerns. Women who have PCOS are more likely to develop insulin resistance, obesity, and type 2 diabetes. The diverse character of PCOS emphasizes the significance of a comprehensive approach to its management and treatment.

Understanding the causes and symptoms of Polycystic Ovary Syndrome (PCOS) is essential for identifying and managing this complicated health problem. PCOS is a complex condition, and while the specific cause is unknown, various risk factors have been discovered.

PCOS causes include:

PCOS has a significant hereditary component, with a greater risk of development among individuals with a family history of the disease. Certain hereditary factors may alter hormonal and metabolic processes, resulting in PCOS.

1. Genetic Predisposition: There is a notable genetic component to PCOS, with a higher likelihood of occurrence among individuals with a family history of the syndrome. Certain genetic factors may influence hormonal and metabolic processes, contributing to the development of PCOS.

2. Insulin Resistance: Insulin resistance plays a significant role in PCOS development. When cells become less responsive to insulin, the body compensates by producing more insulin. Elevated insulin levels can stimulate the ovaries to produce excess androgens, disrupting the normal ovarian function and contributing to the characteristic symptoms of PCOS.

3. Hormonal Imbalances: PCOS is marked by imbalances in reproductive hormones, particularly elevated levels of androgens (male hormones) such as testosterone. This hormonal disruption can affect the regularity of menstrual cycles and lead to the development of ovarian cysts.

PCOS is characterized by hormonal abnormalities, including increased levels of androgens (male hormones) such as testosterone. This hormonal imbalance can interrupt menstrual cycles and contribute to the formation of ovarian cysts.

PCOS symptoms include:

1. **Irregular Menstrual Cycles:** An irregular or missing menstrual cycle is one of the defining signs of PCOS. The hormonal abnormalities associated with PCOS might disturb the normal ovulatory process, affecting menstrual cycle regularity.

2. **Hyperandrogenism:** Excessive androgen levels can cause acne, hirsutism (excessive hair growth, particularly in regions where males generally produce hair), and male-pattern baldness.

3. **Polycystic Ovaries:** As the name implies, PCOS is characterized by the presence of many tiny cysts on the ovaries. These cysts can be seen using imaging techniques such as ultrasonography.

4. **Insulin Resistance and Weight Gain:** Many people with PCOS have insulin resistance, which can contribute to weight gain, particularly around the abdomen. As a result, the hormonal abnormalities associated with PCOS are exacerbated.

5. **Fertility Issues:** PCOS, which causes irregular ovulation, is a prevalent cause of infertility. Managing PCOS is typically an important element of fertility therapy for people trying to conceive.

HOW PCOS IMPACTS YOUR HORMONES

PCOS has a significant impact on hormonal balance, altering the delicate interplay of reproductive hormones and causing a cascade of repercussions across the endocrine system. Understanding how PCOS affects hormones is critical for understanding the complicated mechanisms at work and developing appropriate treatment options.

1. Hyperandrogenism: PCOS is distinguished by increased levels of androgens, sometimes known as male hormones. Androgens are hormones such as testosterone, DHEA, and androstenedione. The increased presence of these hormones can cause symptoms such as acne, hirsutism (excessive hair growth), and male-pattern baldness. Excess androgens also contribute to irregular menstrual periods by interrupting the normal ovulatory process.

2. Insulin Resistance: Insulin resistance is a crucial feature of PCOS, in which the body's cells become less receptive to insulin. Insulin, a hormone generated by the pancreas, is essential for blood sugar regulation. Insulin resistance causes the pancreas to generate extra insulin to compensate in the context of PCOS. Insulin levels that are too high encourage the ovaries to create more androgens, worsening hormonal abnormalities. This insulin resistance also adds to weight gain, which is frequent in PCOS patients.

3. Inhibited Gonadotropin control: PCOS interferes with the proper control of gonadotropins, which are hormones that play an important role in the menstrual cycle. Follicle-stimulating hormone (FSH) and luteinizing hormone (LH) are two important gonadotropins involved in ovarian follicle development and egg release from the ovaries. The equilibrium between FSH and LH is disrupted in PCOS, which contributes to irregular ovulation.

4. Ovarian Dysfunction: Individuals with PCOS frequently have ovarian dysfunction defined by the appearance of many tiny cysts. These cysts form as a result of ovarian follicles failing to develop and release eggs throughout the menstrual cycle. On imaging studies, the concentration of these small follicles adds to the typical look of polycystic ovaries.

Understanding how PCOS impacts hormones lays the groundwork for designing therapies to address the syndrome's unique abnormalities. In the next chapters, we will look at holistic approaches to health, such as plant-based diets, lifestyle changes, and other methods for restoring hormonal balance and increasing general well-being.

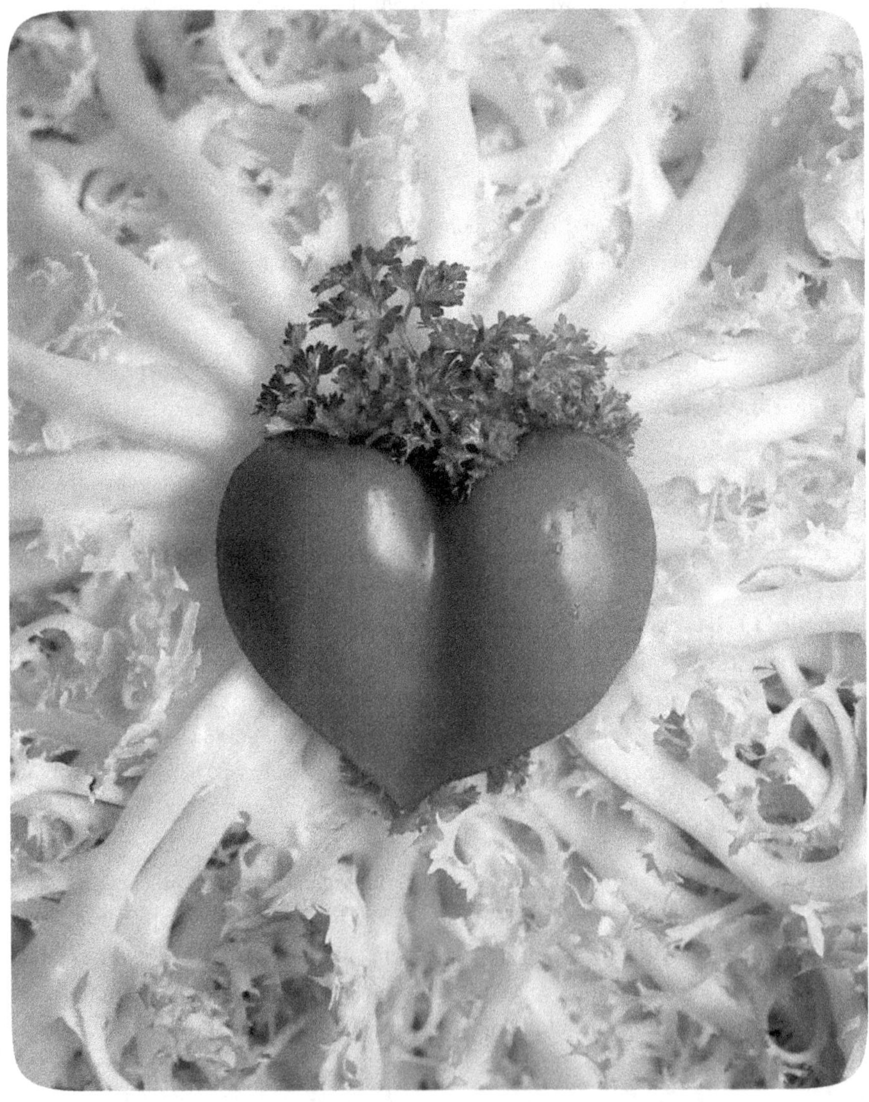

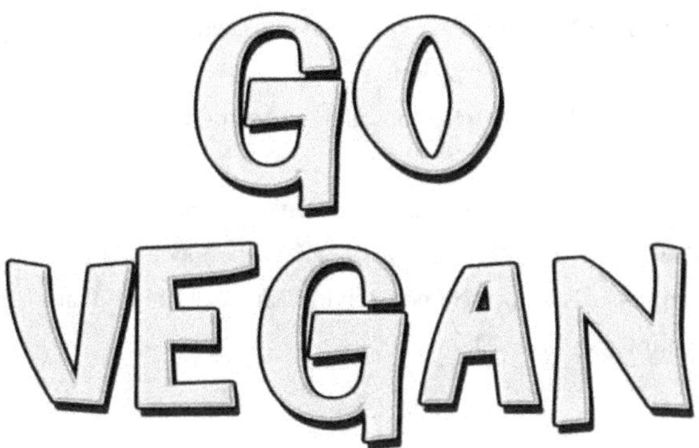

PLANT-BASED DIETS FOR PCOS

For people suffering from Polycystic Ovary Syndrome (PCOS), adopting a plant-based diet may be a transformational and inspiring experience. Plant-based diets, which are high in whole, unprocessed foods produced from plants, have several advantages that are in line with the aims of PCOS therapy.

1. Nutrient Density and entire Foods: Plant-based diets stress the intake of entire, nutrient-dense foods such fruits, vegetables, legumes, whole grains, nuts, and seeds. These foods are high in vitamins, minerals, antioxidants, and fiber, which promote general health while also meeting particular nutritional needs linked with PCOS.

2. Anti-Inflammatory Properties: PCOS is frequently associated with chronic inflammation, which contributes to insulin resistance and hormonal abnormalities. Plant-based diets are anti-inflammatory by nature, with many plant components proven to lower inflammation. Incorporating nutrients like berries, leafy greens, and turmeric into your diet can help your body manage inflammation.

3. Maintaining Stable Blood Sugar Levels: Maintaining stable blood sugar levels is critical for those with PCOS, especially given the prevalence of insulin resistance. Plant-based diets, which are high in complex carbs and fiber, encourage moderate and constant glucose absorption, which helps to reduce blood sugar spikes and crashes.

4. Weight Control: Obesity is a significant issue for those with PCOS, and it can aggravate symptoms. Plant-based diets, when properly organized, can help with weight management and may even help with weight reduction. Furthermore, the emphasis on whole meals helps people feel full, supporting a long-term and healthy approach to weight management.

5. Hormonal Balance: Hormonal balance may be influenced by some plant chemicals, such as phytoestrogens found in soy products. While study on this area is ongoing, adopting a range of plant foods may help with hormonal balance and reproductive health.

6. Gut Health: The gut micro biome is important for general health, including hormone balance. Plant-based diets that are high in fiber feed beneficial gut bacteria, promoting a healthy gut environment. This has the potential to improve metabolism and inflammation, both of which are important in PCOS.

BOOSTING FERTILITY NATURALLY

Adopting natural techniques to fertility enhancement may be both uplifting and successful for people dealing with Polycystic Ovary Syndrome (PCOS). This subchapter digs into holistic fertility-boosting options that take into account the particular problems and concerns connected with PCOS.

1. Hormone Balancing:

Achieving hormonal balance is critical to fertility, and it's especially important for those with PCOS. Natural treatments frequently include lifestyle changes such as stress management, regular exercise, and adequate sleep. These elements contribute to hormonal balance, producing a fertile environment.

2. Nutrient-Rich Diet:

A nutritious and well-balanced diet is essential for fertility. A varied diet rich in fruits, vegetables, whole grains, and lean meats offers important vitamins and minerals that promote reproductive health. Specific nutrients, such as folic acid, omega-3 fatty acids, and antioxidants, play important roles in fertility and can be obtained by food or supplementation.

3. Maintaining a Healthy Weight:

While weight does not entirely influence fertility, obtaining and maintaining a healthy weight can improve reproductive function. A balanced approach to eating and frequent physical activity benefits both general health and fertility in those with PCOS, where weight control is typically a concern.

4. Stress Reduction Methods:

Chronic stress can alter hormonal balance and negatively impact fertility. Stress-reduction strategies like mindfulness, meditation, or yoga might be effective. These activities not only promote mental well-being, but they also stimulate reproductive health.

5. Regular Exercise:

Regular physical exercise has been linked to increased fertility. Exercise aids in the regulation of insulin levels, weight management, and stress reduction. Individualizing training regimens to individual tastes and demands improves long-term success and enjoyment.

6. Ovulation Timing and charting:

Understanding and charting the menstrual cycle, particularly ovulation, is critical for increasing the odds of conception. Identifying fertile times can be aided by a variety of approaches, including ovulation prediction kits and measuring basal body temperature.

7. Natural Supplements:

Certain natural supplements, such as myo-inositol, have showed potential in assisting PCOS patients with fertility. These supplements may aid in the regulation of menstrual cycles, the improvement of ovulatory function, and the enhancement of overall reproductive results. Consultation with a healthcare practitioner is recommended as with any supplement.

WEIGHT LOSS TECHNIQUES

Excess weight can worsen symptoms and contribute to hormone imbalances, thus weight control is generally a major priority for those with PCOS. This subchapter delves into successful and long-term weight loss strategies targeted to the particular issues of PCOS.

1. A Nutrient-Dense and Balanced Diet:

A nutrient-dense and balanced diet is essential for weight management. Concentrate on entire, unprocessed foods such as fruits, vegetables, lean meats, and whole grains. Limiting your intake of processed foods, added sugars, and refined carbs will help you lose weight in a healthy way.

2. Portion Control:

Practicing portion control is essential for calorie management. Paying attention to portion sizes aids in the prevention of overeating and promotes slow, consistent weight reduction. Mindful eating, in which people enjoy and appreciate each meal, can help people become more conscious of hunger and fullness cues.

3. Regular Physical exercise:

Regular physical exercise is essential for general health and weight control. Perform a combination of cardio, strength, and flexibility exercises. To enhance calorie burning and improve metabolic health, tailor the workout regimen to personal tastes and progressively increase intensity.

4. Mindful Eating Practices:

Mindful eating entails paying full attention and being completely present throughout meals. This technique promotes a stronger link to hunger and fullness cues, which helps to reduce emotional or stress-related eating. Mindful eating can help you make healthier food choices and have a better connection with food.

5. Hydration:

Staying hydrated is important for general health and can help you lose weight. Drinking water before meals may aid in appetite management, and drinking water rather than sweetened beverages decreases calorie consumption. Hydration is also important for metabolic function.

6. Excellent Sleep:

Prioritizing excellent sleep is sometimes disregarded in weight-loss conversations. Sleep deprivation can upset hormonal balance, including insulin regulation and hunger hormones. To promote general health and weight reduction goals, aim for 7-9 hours of restful sleep every night.

7. Stress Management:

Chronic stress can lead to weight gain and make it difficult to lose weight. Incorporate stress-reduction strategies such as meditation, deep breathing, or relaxation exercises. These techniques help to maintain hormonal balance and a healthy mentality.

8. Individualized Approach:

Recognize that losing weight is a highly personalized experience. What works for one individual might not work for the next. Experiment with various ways and consider working with healthcare specialists, dietitians, or fitness experts to create a strategy that is tailored to your individual requirements and goals.

Understanding the delicate interplay between insulin and Polycystic Ovary Syndrome (PCOS) is critical for managing and resolving the particular issues faced by this illness. This subchapter investigates the role of insulin in PCOS and solutions for improving insulin function.

1. Insulin Resistance in PCOS:

Insulin is a pancreatic hormone that regulates blood sugar levels. Insulin resistance is a typical occurrence in PCOS. Insulin resistance occurs when the body's cells become less receptive to insulin, resulting in high blood sugar levels.

2. Impact on Hormonal Balance:

Insulin resistance in PCOS has far-reaching consequences on hormonal balance. Elevated insulin levels drive the ovaries to create excess androgens (male hormones), which contributes to the typical symptoms of PCOS, such as irregular menstrual periods, acne, and hirsutism. The altered hormonal balance might increase insulin resistance, generating a feedback cycle.

3. Contribution to Weight Gain:

Insulin resistance is frequently connected with weight gain, particularly in the abdomen area. Excess weight, in turn, can lead to insulin resistance, producing a vicious cycle that can be difficult to overcome. Addressing insulin resistance is critical not just for hormonal balance but also for successful weight control.

4. Importance of Lifestyle Changes:

Lifestyle changes are critical in controlling insulin resistance. Regular physical activity, particularly exercises that promote insulin sensitivity, such as aerobic exercise and strength training, can be quite helpful. Adopting a balanced and nutrient-dense diet, as covered in earlier subchapters, also aids in insulin management.

5. Medication and Supplements:

In some circumstances, healthcare practitioners may prescribe drugs or supplements to treat insulin resistance. Metformin, for example, is a medicine often used to increase insulin sensitivity. Myo-inositol, a naturally occurring substance, has also showed promise in improving insulin action in PCOS patients.

6. Carbohydrate Management:

Because insulin plays such an important role in carbohydrate metabolism, controlling carbohydrate intake is critical. Choosing complex carbs with a low glycemic index will help manage blood sugar levels and minimize insulin sensitivity. This includes eating whole grains, beans, and fiber veggies.

7. Regular testing and Consultation:

People with PCOS, particularly those with insulin resistance, benefit from regular blood sugar testing. Healthcare practitioners can advise on ideal levels and prescribe suitable treatments. Regular discussions with healthcare specialists ensure a tailored strategy to controlling insulin resistance.

Individuals with PCOS can effectively manage insulin resistance by addressing it through a mix of lifestyle changes, medicines if necessary, and dietary changes. This not only helps with hormone balance, but it also promotes general health and well-being.

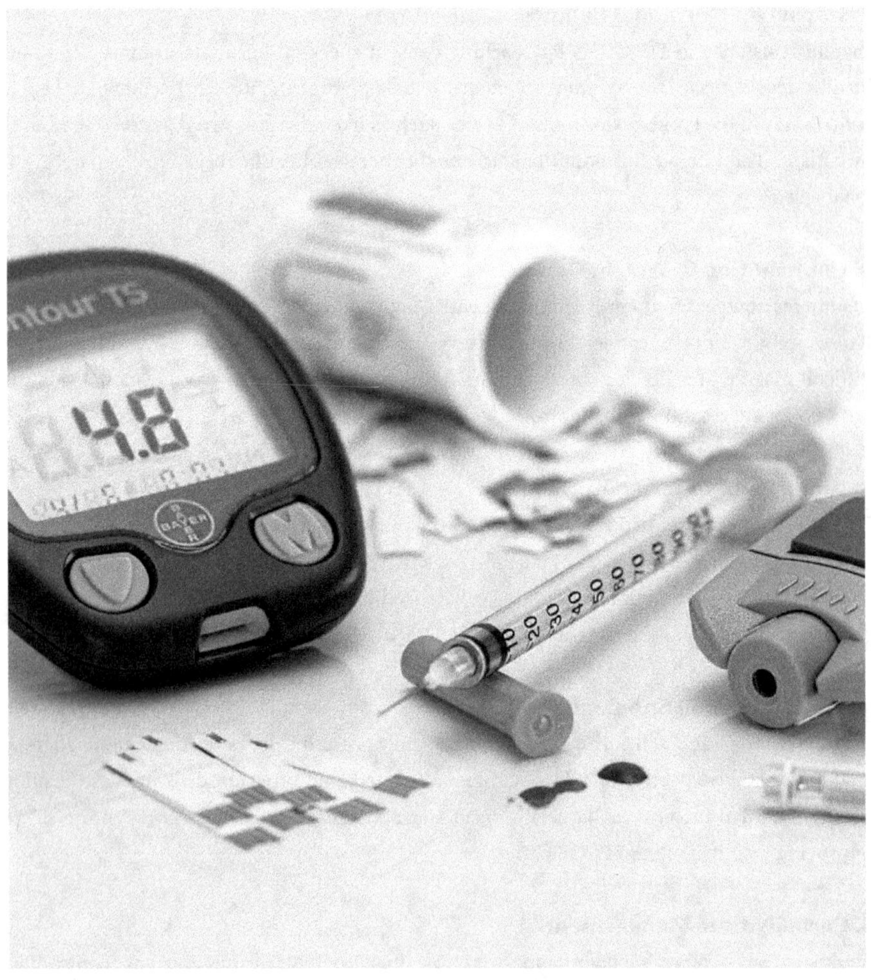

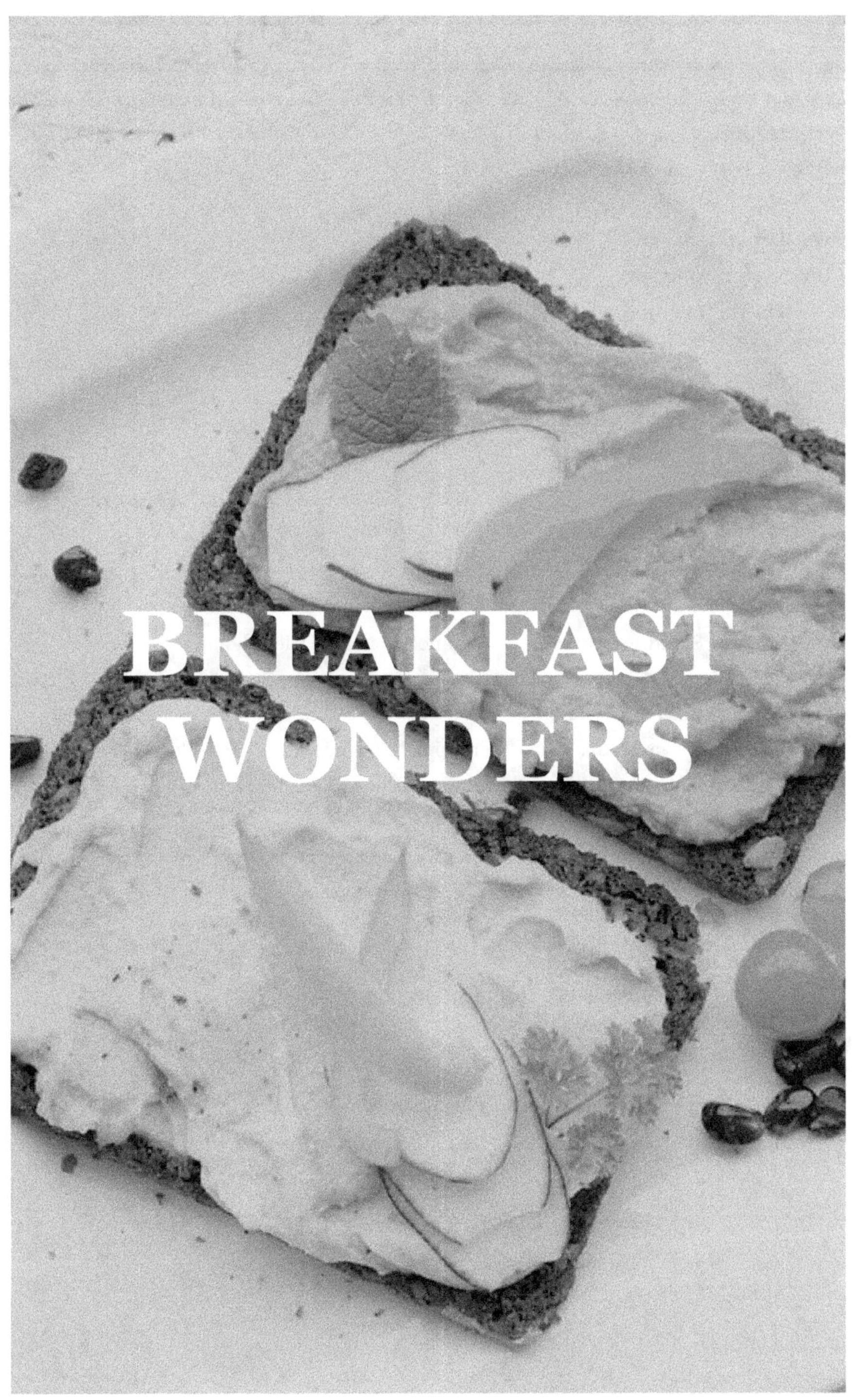
BREAKFAST
WONDERS

With our Green Smoothie Bowl, you can start your day with a rush of freshness. This bowl, packed with nutrient-rich greens and tasty fruits, not only delights your taste senses but also helps you start your day on a positive note.

Prep Time: 10 minutes
Cook Time: 0 minutes
Serves: 1

Ingredients:

- 1 cup spinach leaves, fresh
- 1/2 avocado, ripe
- 1/2 banana, frozen
- 1/2 cup pineapple chunks, frozen
- 1/2 cup almond milk
- 1 tablespoon chia seeds
- Toppings: Sliced strawberries, kiwi, granola, and a drizzle of honey

Step-by-Step Instructions:

1. Blend spinach, avocado, banana, pineapple, and almond milk in a blender.
2. Blend the contents until it is smooth and creamy.
3. Fill a bowl halfway with the smoothie.
4. Top with sliced strawberries, kiwi, granola, and honey drizzle.
5. Chia seeds can be added for an extra nutritious boost.

Nutritional Information:

Calories: 350 | Protein: 8g | Fiber: 15g | Fat: 18g | Carbohydrates: 45g

Pro Tips:

- To add diversity, try various greens such as kale or arugula.
- Adjust the thickness to your liking by adding more or less almond milk.

Our Quinoa and Berry Parfait will take your breakfast routine to the next level. This nutritious blend of quinoa, yogurt, and fresh berries is a delicious way to start the day.

Prep Time: 15 minutes

Cook Time: 15 minutes (quinoa)

Serves: 2

Ingredients:

- 1/2 cup washed quinoa
- 1 cup plain Greek yogurt
- 1 cup berries (strawberries, blueberries, and raspberries)
- 2 teaspoons honey
- 1/4 cup chopped almonds
- 1 tsp vanilla extract

Step-by-Step Instructions:

1. Cook the quinoa as directed on the box and leave aside to cool.
2. Layer quinoa, Greek yogurt, and mixed berries in serving glasses.
3. Drizzle honey over each layer, then top with chopped almonds.
4. Repeat the layering until the glasses are completely full.
5. Finish with a drizzle of vanilla essence.

Nutritional Information:

Calories: 400 | Protein: 20g | Fiber: 8g | Fat: 15g | Carbohydrate: 55g

Pro Tips:

- To add sweetness, use flavored yogurt.
- Make this parfait ahead of time for a simple grab-and-go breakfast.

Try our Avocado Toast Variations for a delicious touch on your daily routine. These Instagram-worthy toasts are a delectable combination of tastes and textures.

Prep Time: 10 minutes

Cook Time: 5 minutes

Serves: 2

Ingredients:

- 2 slices whole wheat bread
- 1 avocado, ripe
- 1 chopped small tomato
- 1 (optional) poached egg
- Season with salt and pepper to taste.
- Red pepper flakes for heat
- For garnish, use fresh cilantro or basil.

Step-by-Step Instructions:

1. Toast the whole-grain bread pieces to the crispiness you choose.
2. Spread the mashed avocado equally on the toasted bread.
3. If preferred, top with sliced tomatoes and a poached egg.
4. Season with salt, pepper, and crushed red pepper flakes to taste.
5. For an added taste boost, garnish with fresh cilantro or basil.

Nutritional Information:

Calories: 300 | Protein: 10g | Fiber: 8g | Fats: 18g | Carbohydrates: 30g

Pro Tips:

- Experiment with different toppings, like as feta cheese or radishes.
- Select a high-quality whole-grain bread for increased nourishment.

Boost your morning energy with this protein-rich Chickpea and Spinach Salad. For a filling breakfast, this substantial salad combines the nutrition of chickpeas, fresh veggies, and a spicy vinaigrette.

Prep Time: 15 minutes

Cook Time: 0 minutes

Serves: 2

Ingredients:

- 1 can (15 oz) washed and drained chickpeas
- 2 cups spinach leaves, fresh
- 1 cup diced cucumber
- 1/2 cup halved cherry tomatoes
- 1/4 cup coarsely sliced red onion 1/4 cup crumbled feta cheese
- 2 tbsp of olive oil
- 1 tbsp. balsamic vinegar
- Season with salt and pepper to taste.

Step-by-Step Instructions:

1. Combine chickpeas, spinach, cucumber, cherry tomatoes, red onion, and feta cheese in a large mixing basin.
2. In a small mixing bowl, combine the olive oil and balsamic vinegar.
3. Toss the salad with the dressing until completely incorporated.
4. Season to taste with salt and pepper.
5. Serve immediately or chill for a quick grab-and-go breakfast.

Nutritional Information:

Calories: 350g | Protein: 12g | Fiber: 10g | Fats: 15g | Carbohydrates: 45g

Pro Tips:

- For an added protein boost, add grilled chicken or tofu.
- Make the dressing ahead of time and keep it separate for a speedy assembling.

Use our Lentil and Vegetable Wrap to wrap up a healthful breakfast. This compact lunch is ideal for folks on the go since it is high in protein, fiber, and a variety of bright vegetables.

Prep Time: 20 minutes

Cook Time: 15 minutes (for lentils)

Serves: 2

Ingredients:

- 1 cup lentils, cooked
- 2 whole-wheat tortillas
- 1/2 cup sliced cherry tomatoes 1/2 cucumber, julienned 1/4 cup thinly sliced red bell pepper
- 1/4 cup crumbled feta cheese
- Hummus (two tablespoons)
- For garnish, use chopped fresh parsley.
- Serve with lemon wedges

Step-by-Step Instructions:

1. Combine cooked lentils, cherry tomatoes, cucumber, red bell pepper, and feta cheese in a mixing bowl.
2. In a dry skillet or microwave, warm the tortillas.
3. Distribute the hummus equally on each tortilla.
4. Fill each tortilla halfway with the lentil and veggie mixture.
5. Fold the sides to make a wrap and garnish with fresh parsley.

Nutritional Information:

Calories: 400g | Protein: 15g | Fiber: 12g | Fats: 10g | Carbohydrates: 60g

Pro Tips:

- Add your favorite vegetables or a sprinkle of tahini for added flavor.
- Make a double batch and split the filling for a quick breakfast throughout the week.

Our Sweet Potato and Kale Bowl will brighten up your morning with brilliant colors and tastes. This antioxidant-rich dish is not only tasty but also a nutritious powerhouse to start the day.

Prep Time: 15 minutes
Cook Time: 20 minutes
Serves: 2

Ingredients:

- 2 medium diced sweet potatoes
- 2 cups destemmed and chopped kale
- 1 tablespoon extra-virgin olive oil
- 1 smoked paprika teaspoon
- Season with salt and pepper to taste.
- 2 eggs (poached or fried, optional)
- 1/4 cup crumbled feta cheese
- Toppings: pumpkin seeds

Step-by-Step Instructions:

1. Preheat the oven to 400 degrees F (200 degrees C).
2. Toss the sweet potato cubes in a bowl with the olive oil, smoked paprika, salt, and pepper.
3. Roast sweet potatoes till golden and soft in the oven.
4. Sauté kale in a skillet until wilted.
5. Arrange roasted sweet potatoes, sautéed kale, poached or fried eggs, and crumbled feta in bowls.
6. To add crunch, garnish with pumpkin seeds.

Nutritional Information:

Calories: 380 | Protein: 15g | Fiber: 8g | Fats: 18g | Carbohydrates: 45g

Pro Tips:

- For added taste, sprinkle with balsamic glaze.
- Make extra roasted sweet potatoes for easy breakfasts throughout the week.

Our Zucchini Noodles with Tomato Sauce are a low-carb take on a classic. This tasty dish is a healthy option that doesn't skimp on flavor.

Prep Time: 15 minutes

Cook Time: 10 minutes

Serves: 2

Ingredients:

- 4 medium spiralized zucchinis
- 1 tablespoon extra virgin olive oil
- 2 minced garlic cloves
- 1 can (14 oz) tomatoes that have been crushed
- 1 tsp. dried oregano
- Optional: 1/2 teaspoon red pepper flakes
- Season with salt and pepper to taste.
- Garnish with fresh basil
- Optional: grated Parmesan cheese

Step-by-Step Instructions:

1. In a skillet, heat the olive oil and sauté the minced garlic until fragrant.
2. Combine the crushed tomatoes, oregano, red pepper flakes (if using), salt, and pepper in a mixing bowl. Cook for 10 minutes.
3. Sauté zucchini noodles in a separate pan until just soft.
4. Serve with tomato sauce and zucchini noodles.
5. Garnish with fresh basil and grated Parmesan cheese, if preferred.

Nutritional Information:

Calories: 220g | Protein: 6g | Fiber: 8g | Fats: 10g | Carbohydrates: 30g

Pro Tips:

- Make the sauce your own by adding your favorite herbs and spices.
- For an added protein boost, add fried shrimp or grilled chicken.

Our Plant-Based Stir-Fry will take your breakfast to the next level. This stir-fry, bursting with bright veggies and tofu, is a flavorful and gratifying way to start your day on a healthy note.

Prep Time: 20 minutes
Cook Time: 15 minutes
Serves: 2

Ingredients:

- 1 cup cubed firm tofu
- 2 teaspoons soy sauce
- 1 tbsp sesame seed oil
- 1 tablespoon minced ginger
- 2 garlic cloves
- 1 bell pepper minced
- 1 cup broccoli florets sliced
- 1 julienned carrot
- 2 sliced green onions
- 2 cups cooked brown rice or quinoa

Step-by-Step Instructions:

1. Tofu should be marinated in soy sauce for 10 minutes in a bowl.
2. In a skillet, heat sesame oil and sauté ginger and garlic until aromatic.
3. Cook the marinated tofu till browned.
4. Add the bell pepper, broccoli, and carrot and mix well. Cook until the veggies are cooked but still crunchy.
5. Toss in cooked brown rice or quinoa and green onions.
6. Serve the plant-based stir-fry immediately.

Nutritional Information:

Calories: 400g | Protein: 20g | Fiber: 8g | Fats: 15g | Carbohydrates: 50g

Pro Tips:

- Drizzle with more soy sauce or a dash of sriracha for more flavor.

Our Almond Energy Bites will revitalize your mornings. These no-bake nibbles are the ideal combination of nuts, seeds, and sweetness for a quick and healthful breakfast or snack.

Prep Time: 15 minutes
Cook Time: 0 minutes (no-bake)
Serves: Makes 12 bites

Ingredients:

- 1 cup raw almonds
- 1 pound rolled oats
- 1 tablespoon chia seeds
- 1 tablespoon almond butter
- 1 tablespoon honey or maple syrup
- 1 tsp vanilla extract
- 1 teaspoon salt
- (Optional) shredded coconut for rolling

Step-by-Step Instructions:

1. Combine almonds, rolled oats, and chia seeds in a food processor. Pulse until the mixture is finely minced.
2. Combine almond butter, honey or maple syrup, vanilla extract, and a touch of salt in a mixing bowl. Process the ingredients until it comes together.
3. Scoop out little amounts and shape into bite-sized balls.
4. Roll the energy bites in shredded coconut if desired for extra texture.
5. Allow at least 30 minutes for chilling before serving.

Nutritional Information:

Calories: 100g (per bite) | Protein: 3g | Fiber: 2g | Fats: 7g | Carbohydrates: 8g

Pro Tips:

- Add your favorite nuts or seeds to make it your own.
- Refrigerate in an airtight container for an easy grab-and-go alternative.

Enjoy a relaxing start to your day with our Herbal Infusions for Hormonal Balance. These delectable infusions not only provide warmth and comfort, but also include herbs renowned for their potential hormonal-balancing qualities.

Prep Time: 5 minutes

Cook Time: 5 minutes

Serves: 2

Ingredients:

- 1 tablespoon dried chamomile flowers
- 1 tablespoon dried red clover
- 1 tablespoon dried spearmint leaves
- 2 cups hot water
- Optional honey or lemon

Step-by-Step Instructions:

1. Chamomile flowers, red clover, and spearmint leaves should be combined in a teapot or infuser.
2. Pour boiling water over the herbs and soak for 5 minutes.
3. Pour the infusion into mugs.
4. If desired, sweeten with honey or add a splash of lemon juice.
5. Enjoy the herbal infusion for a peaceful and balanced morning routine.

Nutritional Information:

Calories: 0 | Antioxidants: High | Beneficial Compounds: Chamomile, red clover, and spearmint are known for their potential hormonal-balancing properties.

Pro Tips:

- To add diversity, use lavender or nettle.
- Sip gently and deliberately, enjoying the relaxing benefits of herbal infusions.

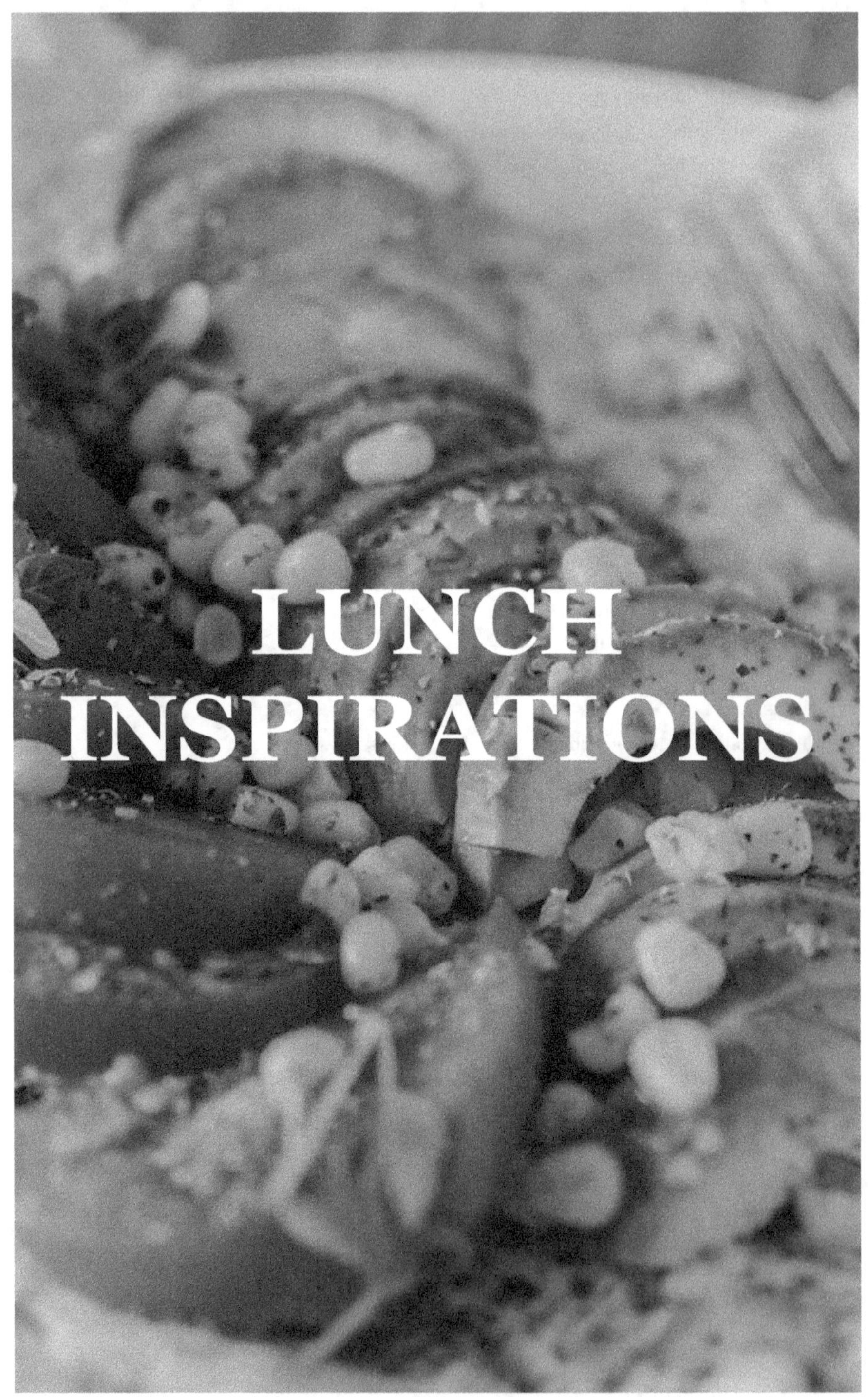
LUNCH
INSPIRATIONS

Upgrade your lunch with this protein-rich Chickpea and Spinach Salad. This rich and tasty salad is not only filling, but also a healthful alternative to keep you energized throughout the day.

Prep Time: 15 minutes
Cook Time: 0 minutes
Serves: 2

Ingredients:

- 1 can (15 oz) chickpeas, drained and rinsed
- 2 cup fresh spinach leaves
- 1 cucumber, diced
- Halved 1/2 cup cherry tomatoes
- 1/4 cup coarsely diced red onion 1/4 cup crumbled feta cheese
- 2 tablespoons olive oil
- 1 tablespoon balsamic vinegar
- To taste, season with salt and pepper.

Step-by-Step Instructions:

1. Combine the chickpeas, spinach, cucumber, cherry tomatoes, red onion, and feta cheese in a large mixing basin.
2. Whisk together the olive oil and balsamic vinegar in a small mixing bowl.
3. Drizzle the dressing over the salad and stir until fully incorporated.
4. Season with salt and pepper, to taste.
5. Serve immediately or chill for a refreshing and nutrient-dense lunch.

Nutritional Information:

Calories: 350g | Protein: 12g | Fiber: 10g | Fats: 15g | Carbohydrates: 45g

Pro Tips:

- Add grilled chicken or tofu for a protein boost.
- Make the dressing ahead of time and keep it separately for easy assembling.

Our Lentil and Vegetable Wrap makes a filling lunch. This compact lunch is ideal for individuals on the go, since it contains plant-based protein and a mix of bright vegetables.

Prep Time: 20 minutes

Cook Time: 15 minutes (for lentils)

Serves: 2

Ingredients:

- 1 cup lentils, cooked
- 2 whole-wheat tortillas
- 1/2 cup sliced cherry tomatoes
- 1/2 cucumber
- Julienned 1/4 cup thinly sliced red bell pepper
- 1/4 cup crumbled feta cheese
- Hummus (two tablespoons)
- For garnish, use chopped fresh parsley.
- Serve with lemon wedges

Step-by-Step Instructions:

1. Combine cooked lentils, cherry tomatoes, cucumber, red bell pepper, and feta cheese in a mixing bowl.
2. In a dry skillet or microwave, warm the tortillas.
3. Distribute the hummus equally on each tortilla.
4. Fill each tortilla halfway with the lentil and veggie mixture.
5. Fold the sides and garnish with fresh parsley to make a lovely wrap.

Nutritional Information:

Calories: 400g Protein: 15g | Fiber: 12g | Fats: 10g | Carbohydrates: 60g

Pro Tips:

- Add your favorite vegetables or a sprinkle of tahini for added flavor.
- Make a double batch and split the filling for a fast lunch throughout the week.

Our soothing Minestrone Soup will warm up your lunchtime. This substantial soup is a filling and delicious noon meal, packed with veggies, beans, and flavorful broth.

Prep Time: 20 minutes
Cook Time: 30 minutes
Serves: 4

Ingredients:

- 1 tablespoon extra-virgin olive oil
- 1 onion, diced 2 carrots
- Sliced 2 celery stalks,
- Chopped 3 garlic cloves, minced
- 1 can (15 oz) chopped tomatoes
- 1 can (15 oz) drained and washed kidney beans
- 4 cups veggie broth
- 1 cup tiny pasta (for example, ditalini or elbow)
- 1 diced zucchini
- 1 cup chopped green beans
- 1 tsp. dried oregano
- Season with salt and pepper to taste.
- For garnish, use chopped fresh basil.
- Parmesan cheese, grated, for serving

Step-by-Step Instructions:

1. Warm the olive oil in a large saucepan over medium heat.
2. Cook until the onion, carrots, and celery are softened.
3. After adding the garlic, cook for another minute.
4. Combine chopped tomatoes, kidney beans, vegetable broth, pasta, zucchini, green beans, oregano, salt, and pepper in a mixing bowl.
5. Bring to a boil, then lower to a low heat and cook until the pasta and veggies are cooked.
6. Serve hot, garnished with fresh basil and topped with grated Parmesan cheese.

Nutritional Information:

Calories: 300g | Protein: 10g | Fiber: 8g | Fats: 8g | Carbohydrates: 45g

Pro Tips:

- Add your favorite veggies or a handful of spinach for added greens.

Our Quinoa and Black Bean Salad is bursting with flavor. This salad is a healthful and tasty alternative for a full lunch, packed with protein, fiber, and a spicy dressing.

Prep Time: 15 minutes
Cook Time: 15 minutes (for quinoa)
Serves: 3

Ingredients:

- 1 cup washed quinoa
- 1 can (15 oz) washed and drained black beans
- 1 cup fresh or frozen corn kernels
- 1 chopped red bell pepper
- 1/4 cup coarsely chopped red onion
- 1/4 cup chopped cilantro
- 1 diced avocado
- 2 limes juice
- 2 tbsp of olive oil
- Season with salt and pepper to taste.

Step-by-Step Instructions:

1. Cook the quinoa as directed on the box and leave aside to cool.
2. Combine cooked quinoa, black beans, corn, red bell pepper, red onion, cilantro, and avocado in a large mixing basin.
3. In a small mixing bowl, combine the lime juice, olive oil, salt, and pepper.
4. Toss the salad with the dressing until completely incorporated.
5. Serve chilled, topped with more cilantro.

Nutritional Information:
Calories: 380g | Protein: 15g | Fiber: 12g | Fats: 15g | Carbohydrates: 50g

Pro Tips:

- For an added kick, add chopped tomatoes or jalapeos.
- For a fast and delicious lunch, prepare the salad the night before.

Refresh yourself with our Detoxifying Cucumber Gazpacho. This chilled soup, filled with cucumber and mint freshness, is an ideal light lunch alternative for hot days.

Prep Time: 15 minutes
Cook Time: 0 minutes
Serves: 4

Ingredients:

- 3 big peeled and sliced cucumbers
- 1 green bell pepper
- Diced 1/2 red onion
- Diced 2 garlic cloves
- Minced 1/4 cup fresh dill
- Minced 1/4 cup fresh mint
- Minced 2 cups vegetable broth
- 1 tablespoon white wine vinegar
- Season with salt and pepper to suit.
- Garnish with Greek yogurt (optional).

Step-by-Step Instructions:

1. In a blender, combine cucumbers, green bell pepper, red onion, garlic, dill, mint, vegetable broth, and white wine vinegar.
2. Blend until smooth.
3. Season with salt and pepper to taste.
4. Allow at least 2 hours before serving to chill.
5. Garnish with a dollop of Greek yogurt if desired.

Nutritional Information:

Calories: 70g | Protein: 2g | Fiber: 3g | Fats: 1g | Carbohydrates: 15g

Pro Tips:

- Serve the gazpacho in chilled bowls for an extra refreshing experience.
- Experiment with additional herbs like basil or cilantro for different flavor profiles.

Our Quinoa and Berry Salad provides a blast of freshness. This salad is a delicious and nutritious lunch alternative, packed with the benefits of quinoa, mixed berries, and a zesty vinaigrette.

Prep Time: 15 minutes

Cook Time: 15 minutes (for quinoa)

Serves: 3

Ingredients:

- 1 cup washed quinoa
- 1 cup berries (strawberries, blueberries, and raspberries)
- 1/4 cup crumbled feta cheese
- 1/4 cup chopped fresh mint
- 2 tbsp. balsamic vinaigrette
- 1 tablespoon extra-virgin olive oil
- Season with salt and pepper to taste.
- Optional: 1/4 cup chopped walnuts

Step-by-Step Instructions:

1. Cook the quinoa as directed on the box and leave aside to cool.
2. Combine cooked quinoa, mixed berries, feta cheese, and fresh mint in a large mixing basin.
3. In a small mixing bowl, combine the balsamic vinaigrette, olive oil, salt, and pepper.
4. Drizzle the dressing over the salad and gently mix to combine.
5. For added crunch, garnish with chopped walnuts.

Nutritional Information:

Calories: 350g | Protein: 10g | Fiber: 8g | Fats: 15g | Carbohydrates: 50g

Pro Tips:

- For an added protein boost, add grilled chicken or tofu.
- Make a bigger batch and keep it in the refrigerator for fast and refreshing lunches.

Enjoy a hearty and filling lunch with our Stuffed Bell Peppers. This colorful and healthful dish is filled with a savory blend of quinoa, black beans, and veggies.

Prep Time: 20 minutes

Cook Time: 25 minutes

Serves: 4

Ingredients:

- 4 big bell peppers, peeled and halved
- 1 cup cooked quinoa
- 1 can (15 oz) washed and drained black beans
- 1 cup fresh or frozen corn kernels
- 1 cup chopped cherry tomatoes
- 1/2 coarsely chopped red onion
- 1 tablespoon cumin
- 1 tsp. chili powder
- Half-cup crumbled cheddar cheese
- Chopped fresh cilantro for garnish
- Serving slices of lime

Step-by-Step Instructions:

1. Preheat the oven to 375 degrees F (190 degrees C).
2. Combine cooked quinoa, black beans, corn, cherry tomatoes, red onion, cumin, and chili powder in a mixing bowl.
3. Fill each half of a bell pepper with the quinoa mixture.
4. Shredded cheddar cheese on top.
5. Bake the peppers for 25 minutes, or until tender.
6. Serve with lime wedges and garnished with fresh cilantro.

Nutritional Information:

Calories: 320g | Protein: 12g | Fiber: 10g | Fats: 10g | Carbohydrates: 45g

Pro Tips:

- For a more lively display, experiment with different colored bell peppers.
- Drizzle with spicy sauce for a little more heat.

Our Zucchini and Chickpea Patties are a protein-packed and tasty lunch option. These delicious patties are an excellent way to include vegetables and plant-based protein in your noon meal.

Prep Time: 25 minutes
Cook Time: 15 minutes
Serves: 3

Ingredients:

- 1 can (15 oz) 2 medium zucchinis
- Grated drained and washed chickpeas
- 1 pound breadcrumbs
- 1/4 cup coarsely chopped red onion
- 2 minced garlic cloves
- 1 tablespoon cumin
- 1 paprika teaspoon
- Season with salt and pepper to taste.
- 2 tbsp of olive oil
- For serving, use Greek yogurt or tahini sauce.

Step-by-Step Instructions:

1. Squeeze excess water from shredded zucchinis in a clean kitchen towel.
2. Combine zucchini, chickpeas, breadcrumbs, red onion, garlic, cumin, paprika, salt, and pepper in a food processor. Pulse until everything is properly blended.
3. Make patties out of the mixture.
4. In a pan, heat the olive oil and fry the patties until brown on both sides.
5. Serve immediately with a dollop of Greek yogurt or a splash of tahini sauce.

Nutritional Information:
Calories: 280g | Protein: 10g | Fiber: 8g | Fats: 10g | Carbohydrates: 40g

Pro Tips:

- Make the patties your own by adding your favorite herbs and spices.
- For a new touch, serve on a whole-grain bread or lettuce wraps.

MEDITERRANEAN QUINOA BOWL

Our vivid and tasty Mediterranean Quinoa Bowl will transport your taste senses to the Mediterranean. This bowl is a wonderful and nutritious lunch alternative, packed with colorful vegetables, olives, and a spicy dressing.

Prep Time: 20 minutes
Cook Time: 15 minutes (for quinoa)
Serves: 3

Ingredients:

- 1 cup rinsed quinoa
- 1 cup cherry tomatoes
- Halved 1 cucumber
- Diced 1/2 cup pitted and sliced Kalamata olives
- 1/4 cup finely sliced red onion
- 1/4 cup crumbled feta cheese
- For garnish, use chopped fresh parsley.
- 2 tbsp of olive oil
- 1 tbsp. red wine vinegar
- 1 tsp. dried oregano
- Season with salt and pepper to taste.

Step-by-Step Instructions:

1. Cook the quinoa as directed on the box and leave aside to cool.
2. Combine cooked quinoa, cherry tomatoes, cucumber, Kalamata olives, red onion, and feta cheese in a large mixing bowl.
3. Whisk together olive oil, red wine vinegar, dried oregano, salt, and pepper in a small bowl.
4. Drizzle the dressing over the quinoa and gently mix.
5. Serve cold, garnished with fresh parsley.

Nutritional Information:

Calories: 330g | Protein: 10g | Fiber: 8g | Fats: 15g | Carbohydrates: 45g

Pro Tips:

- For a protein boost, add grilled chicken or shrimp.
- Make extra to have on hand for a fast and refreshing lunch throughout the week.

Enjoy a nutrient-dense lunch with our Sweet Potato and Chickpea Buddha Bowl. This bright and nutritious bowl is a wonderful blend of flavors and textures, giving a filling and fulfilling lunch.

Prep Time: 25 minutes

Cook Time: 30 minutes

Serves: 3

Ingredients:

- 1 can (15 oz) sweet potatoes, diced chickpeas, washed and drained
- 1 tbsp olive oil
- 1 teaspoon cumin
- 1 teaspoon smoked paprika
- Season with salt and pepper to taste
- 2 cups cooked quinoa
- 1 avocado, sliced
- 1 cup shredded red cabbage
- 1/4 cup tahini sauce
- Sesame seeds for garnish

Step-by-Step Instructions:

1. Preheat the oven to 400°F (200°C).
2. Toss sweet potatoes and chickpeas with olive oil, cumin, smoked paprika, salt, and pepper.
3. Roast until the sweet potatoes are soft and the chickpeas are crunchy.
4. Assemble bowls with cooked quinoa, roasted sweet potatoes and chickpeas, avocado slices, and shredded red cabbage.
5. Drizzle with tahini sauce and sprinkle with sesame seeds to serve.

Nutritional Information:

Calories: 420g | Protein: 15g | Fiber: 12g | Fats: 18g | Carbohydrates: 55g

Pro Tips:

- Make it your own by adding your favorite roasted veggies.
- Make a double batch for meal prep and enjoy Buddha bowls throughout the week.

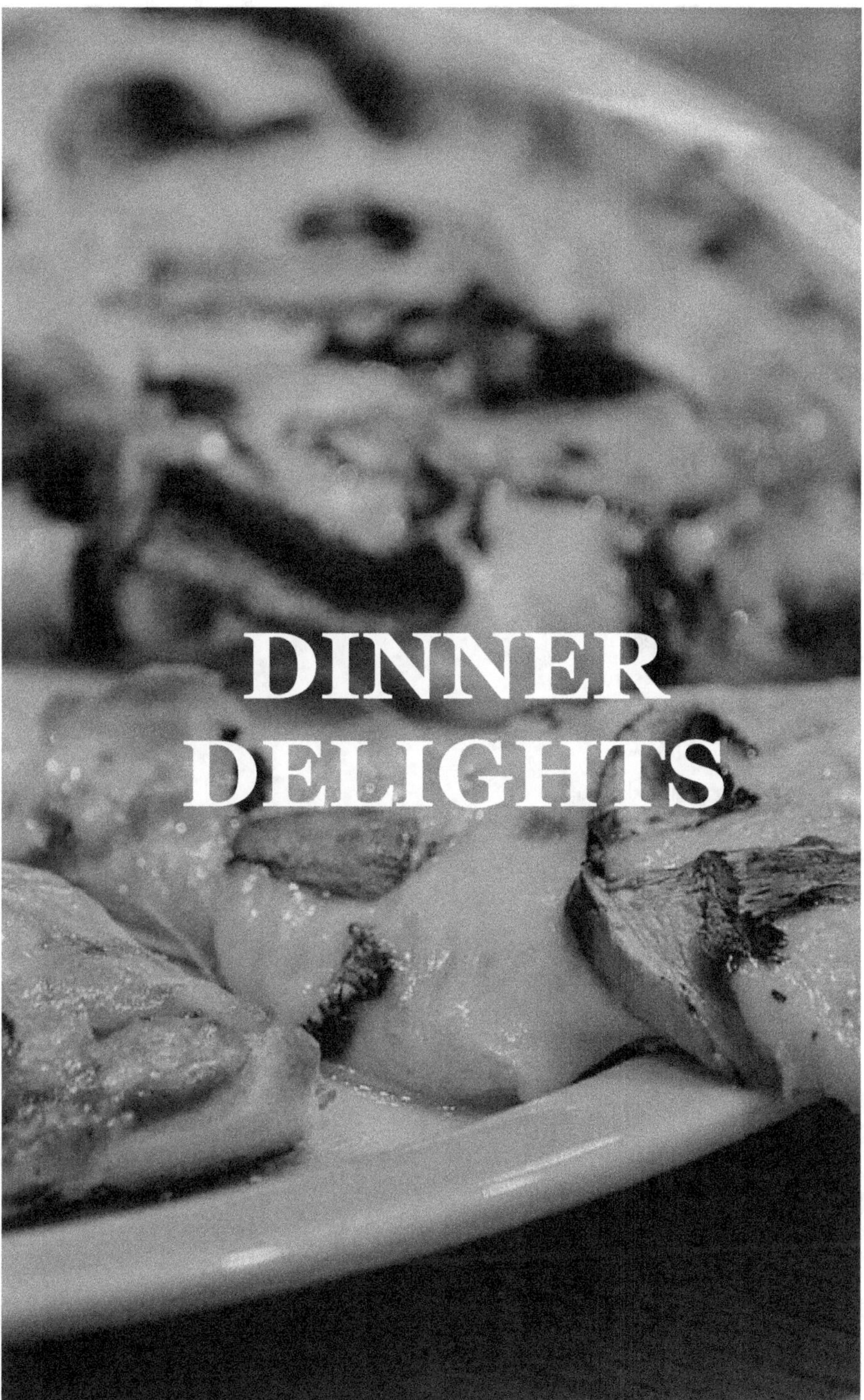

DINNER DELIGHTS

Our Plant-Based Stir-Fry will take your meal to the next level. This stir-fry is a quick and nutritious alternative for a wonderful evening supper, bursting with colorful veggies, tofu, and a rich sauce.

Prep Time: 20 minutes

Cook Time: 15 minutes

Serves: 4

Ingredients:

- 1 firm tofu block, pressed and cubed
- 2 cups florets broccoli
- 1 sliced bell pepper
- 1 julienned carrot
- 1 pound snap peas
- 1 tablespoon soy sauce
- 2 tbsp sesame seed oil
- 1 teaspoon maple syrup
- 1 teaspoon cornstarch
- 2 minced garlic cloves
- 1 tablespoon grated ginger
- Sesame seeds for decoration
- Sliced green onions for garnish
- Brown rice, cooked and ready to serve

Step-by-Step Instructions:

1. To prepare the sauce, combine soy sauce, sesame oil, maple syrup, cornstarch, garlic, and ginger in a mixing bowl.
2. Sauté tofu in a large pan or wok until brown. Take out and set aside.
3. In the same pan, stir-fry broccoli, bell pepper, carrot, and snap peas.
4. Return the fried tofu to the pan and pour the sauce over it.
5. Toss everything together until evenly coated and cooked through.
6. Serve with sesame seeds and sliced green onions on top of cooked brown rice.

Nutritional Information:

Calories: 350g | Protein: 15g | Fiber: 8g | Fats: 12g | Carbohydrates: 45g

Savor a standard with a plant-based twist—our Spaghetti with Lentil Bolognese. This filling and delicious dish is a comfortable choice for a full dinner that's rich in protein and nutrients.

Prep Time: 15 minutes
Cook Time: 30 minutes
4 people

Ingredients::

- 2 cups cooked lentils
- 1 tablespoon olive oil
- 1 onion, finely chopped
- 2 carrots, diced
- 2 celery stalks, chopped
- 3 cloves garlic, minced
- 1 can (15 oz) crushed tomatoes
- 1/2 cup tomato paste
- 1 teaspoon dried oregano
- 1 teaspoon dried basil
- Salt and pepper to taste
- 1 pound whole-grain spaghetti
- Fresh basil, chopped, for garnish
- Vegan Parmesan cheese for serving

Step-by-Step Instructions:

1. In a big pot, heat olive oil and sauté onion, carrots, and celery until softened.
2. Add garlic and cook for an additional minute.
3. Stir in cooked lentils, crushed tomatoes, tomato paste, oregano, basil, salt, and pepper.
4. Simmer the sauce for 20-25 minutes, turning occasionally.
5. Cook spaghetti according to package directions.
6. Serve the lentil Bolognese over cooked spaghetti, topped with fresh basil and veggie Parmesan.

Nutritional Information:

Calories: 400|Protein: 18g | Fiber: 12g | Fats: 8g | Carbohydrates: 60g

Pro Tips:

- Add a splash of red wine to the sauce for extra depth of flavor.

Take your taste buds on a trip with our Chickpea and Spinach Curry. This tasty and aromatic curry is a great plant-based choice for a filling and healthy dinner.

Prep Time: 20 minutes

Cook Time: 25 minutes

Serves: 4

Ingredients:

- 2 cans (15 oz each) chickpeas, drained and washed
- 1 tablespoon coconut oil
- 1 onion, finely chopped
- 3 cloves garlic, minced
- 1 tablespoon ginger, grated
- 2 tablespoons curry powder
- 1 teaspoon crushed cumin
- 1 teaspoon chopped coriander
- 1/2 teaspoon turmeric
- 1 can (14 oz) diced tomatoes
- 1 can (14 oz) coconut milk
- 4 cups fresh spinach leaves
- Salt and pepper to taste
- Cooked brown rice for serving
- Fresh cilantro, chopped, for garnish

Step-by-Step Instructions:

1. In a big pan, heat coconut oil and sauté onion, garlic, and ginger until softened.
2. Add curry powder, cumin, coriander, and turmeric. Stir well.
3. Pour in diced tomatoes and coconut milk, bringing the mixture to a boil.
4. Add chickpeas and cook for 15 minutes, allowing flavors to meld.
5. Add fresh spinach and cook until wilted.
6. Season with salt and pepper and serve over cooked brown rice, topped with fresh cilantro.

Nutritional Information:

Calories: 420g | Protein: 15g | Fiber: 12g | Fats: 15g | Carbohydrates: 55g

Indulge in a gourmet dinner with our Stuffed Portobello Mushrooms. Filled with a savory mixture of quinoa, vegetables, and herbs, these mushrooms are a delightful and satisfying option for a plant-based evening.

Prep Time: 20 minutes

Cook Time: 25 minutes

Serves: 3

Ingredients:

- 6 big Portobello mushrooms, tips removed
- 1 cup quinoa, cooked
- 1 tablespoon olive oil
- 1 onion, finely chopped 2 cloves garlic, minced 1 bell pepper, diced 1 zucchini, diced 1 cup cherry tomatoes, halved 1/4 cup fresh basil, chopped 1/4 cup vegan mozzarella cheese, shredded
- Salt and pepper to taste
- Balsamic glaze for drizzling
- Fresh parsley, chopped, for garnish

Step-by-Step Instructions:

1. Preheat the oven to 375°F (190°C).
2. Place Portobello mushrooms on a baking sheet.
3. In a pan, heat olive oil and sauté onion, garlic, bell pepper, and zucchini until softened.
4. In a bowl, mix cooked quinoa, sautéed vegetables, cherry tomatoes, basil, and vegan mozzarella.
5. Stuff each Portobello mushroom with the quinoa mixture.
6. Bake in the oven for 20-25 minutes or until mushrooms are soft.
7. Drizzle with balsamic glaze and garnish with fresh parsley before serving.

Nutritional Information:

Calories: 380g | Protein: 12g | Fiber: 10g | Fats: 10g | Carbohydrates: 55g

Pro Tips:

- Experiment with different herbs and spices for varied taste combinations.
- Serve over a bed of arugula for a refreshing twist.

Enjoy a light and tasty dinner with our Zucchini Noodles with Tomato Sauce. This low-carb and nutrient-packed food are not only delicious but also a cool choice for a guilt-free evening meal.

Prep Time: 15 minutes

Cook Time: 15 minutes

Serves: 2

Ingredients:

- 4 big zucchinis, spiralized
- 2 tablespoons olive oil
- 3 cloves garlic, minced
- 1 can (15 oz) crushed tomatoes
- 1 teaspoon dried oregano
- 1 teaspoon dried basil
- Salt and pepper to taste
- Red pepper flakes for heat (optional)
- Vegan Parmesan cheese for serving
- Fresh basil, chopped, for garnish

Step-by-Step Instructions:

1. In a pan, heat olive oil and sauté garlic until fragrant.
2. Add crushed tomatoes, oregano, basil, salt, and pepper. Simmer for 10 minutes.
3. In a different pan, sauté zucchini noodles until just soft.
4. Toss zucchini noodles with tomato sauce, ensuring they are well covered.
5. Serve hot, topped with red pepper flakes, veggie Parmesan, and fresh basil.

Nutritional Information:

Calories: 250g | Protein: 8g | Fiber: 10g | Fats: 12g | Carbohydrates: 35g

Pro Tips:

- Customize with extra veggies or protein of your choice.
- Top with nutritional yeast for a cheesy taste without dairy.

Experience a symphony of flavors with our Vegan Stuffed Bell Peppers. Filled with a savory blend of quinoa, black beans, and spices, these stuffed peppers are a satisfying and wholesome addition to your dinner table.

Prep Time: 25 minutes
Cook Time: 30 minutes
Serves: 4

Ingredients:

- 4 large bell peppers, halved and seeds removed
- 1 cup quinoa, cooked
- 1 can (15 oz) black beans, drained and rinsed
- 1 cup corn kernels (fresh or frozen)
- 1 cup diced tomatoes
- 1/2 red onion, finely chopped
- 1 teaspoon cumin
- 1 teaspoon chili powder
- 1/2 teaspoon smoked paprika
- Salt and pepper to taste
- Salsa for topping
- Fresh cilantro, chopped, for garnish

Step-by-Step Instructions:

1. Preheat the oven to 375°F (190°C).
2. In a bowl, combine cooked quinoa, black beans, corn, diced tomatoes, red onion, cumin, chili powder, smoked paprika, salt, and pepper.
3. Fill each bell pepper half with the quinoa mixture.
4. Place the stuffed peppers in a baking dish.
5. Bake for 25-30 minutes or until peppers are tender.
6. Top with salsa and fresh cilantro before serving.

Nutritional Information:

Calories: 320g | Protein: 12g | Fiber: 10g | Fats: 8g | Carbohydrates: 50g

Pro Tips:

- Drizzle with vegan cheese sauce for an extra indulgence.
- Serve over a bed of greens for a lighter option.

Wrap up your day with our hearty Lentil and Vegetable Wrap. Bursting with protein-packed lentils, colorful veggies, and a zesty tahini sauce, this wrap is a delicious and convenient dinner option.

Prep Time: 20 minutes

Cook Time: 15 minutes

Serves: 3

Ingredients:

- 1 cup dry green or brown lentils, cooked
- 1 tablespoon olive oil
- 1 red bell pepper, sliced
- 1 yellow bell pepper, sliced
- 1 zucchini, julienned
- 1 carrot, julienned
- 1/2 red onion, thinly sliced
- 1 teaspoon ground cumin
- 1 teaspoon smoked paprika
- Salt and pepper to taste
- 3 whole-grain wraps
- Tahini sauce for drizzling
- Fresh parsley, chopped, for garnish

Step-by-Step Instructions:

1. In a pan, heat olive oil and sauté bell peppers, zucchini, carrot, and red onion until tender.
2. Add cooked lentils, ground cumin, smoked paprika, salt, and pepper. Stir well.
3. Warm the whole-grain wraps in a dry skillet or microwave.
4. Spoon the lentil and vegetable mixture onto each wrap.
5. Drizzle with tahini sauce and sprinkle with fresh parsley.
6. Fold the wraps and serve immediately.

Nutritional Information:

Calories: 350g | Protein: 15g | Fiber: 8g | Fats: 10g | Carbohydrates: 50g

Pro Tips:

- Add avocado slices for creaminess.
- Serve with a side of mixed greens or a cucumber salad.

Nourish your body with our Sweet Potato and Kale Bowl—a perfect blend of roasted sweet potatoes, sautéed kale, and a spicy tahini dressing. This bowl is a delicious and healthy dinner choice.

Prep Time: 25 minutes
Cook Time: 30 minutes
Serves: 3

Ingredients:

- 2 large sweet potatoes, cubed 1 bunch kale, stems removed and chopped
- 2 tablespoons olive oil
- 1 teaspoon smoked paprika
- 1/2 teaspoon garlic powder
- Salt and pepper to taste
- 1 cup cooked quinoa
- 1/4 cup tahini
- 2 tablespoons lemon juice
- 2 tablespoons water
- 1 tablespoon maple syrup
- Sesame seeds for garnish

Step-by-Step Instructions:

1. Preheat the oven to 400°F (200°C).
2. Toss sweet potatoes with olive oil, smoked paprika, garlic powder, salt, and pepper.
3. Roast in the oven until sweet potatoes are soft.
4. In a pan, sauté chopped kale until limp.
5. In a small bowl, mix together tahini, lemon juice, water, and maple syrup to make the dressing.
6. Assemble bowls with cooked quinoa, roasted sweet potatoes, sautéed kale, and drizzle with tahini dressing.
7. Garnish with sesame seeds before serving.

Nutritional Information:

Calories: 380g | Protein: 10g | Fiber: 10g | Fats: 15g | Carbohydrates: 55g

Pro Tips:

- Add a pinch of nutritional yeast for a cheesy taste.
- Swap kale for spinach or another leafy green.

Warm your soul with our hearty Minestrone Soup. Packed with a mix of veggies, beans, and pasta, this warm soup is a delightful and healthy choice for a cozy dinner.

Prep Time: 20 minutes

Cook Time: 35 minutes

Serves: 6

Ingredients:

- 1 tablespoon olive oil
- 2 carrots, 2 chopped celery stalks, 3 diced garlic cloves, 1 minced can (15 oz) cannellini beans, drained and washed
- 1 can (15 oz) diced tomatoes
- 1 zucchini, diced
- 1 cup green beans, chopped
- 1 cup small pasta (elbow, ditalini, or similar)
- 1 teaspoon dried oregano
- 1 teaspoon dried basil
- Salt and pepper to taste
- 6 cups vegetable broth
- Fresh parsley, chopped, for garnish
- Vegan Parmesan for serving

Step-by-Step Instructions:

1. In a big pot, heat olive oil and sauté onion, carrots, celery, and garlic until softened.
2. Add cannellini beans, diced tomatoes, zucchini, green beans, pasta, oregano, basil, salt, and pepper.
3. Pour in vegetable broth and bring to a simmer.
4. Cook until pasta and veggies are soft.
5. Garnish with fresh parsley and serve hot with a sprinkle of veggie Parmesan.

Nutritional Information:

Calories: 280g | Protein: 10g | Fiber: 8g | Fats: 6g | Carbohydrates: 45g

Pro Tips:

- Make a big batch and freeze for quick, comforting meals.
- Serve with fresh whole-grain bread for a full experience.

QUINOA AND BLACK BEAN SALAD

Delight in the freshness of our Quinoa and Black Bean Salad. Packed with protein-rich quinoa, black beans, and a zesty lime dressing, this salad is a refreshing and satisfying option for a light yet fulfilling dinner.

Prep Time: 20 minutes
Cook Time: 15 minutes (for quinoa)
Serves: 4

Ingredients:

- 1 cup quinoa, rinsed
- 1 can (15 oz) black beans, drained and rinsed
- 1 cup corn kernels (fresh or frozen)
- 1 red bell pepper, diced
- 1/4 cup red onion, finely chopped
- 1/4 cup fresh cilantro, chopped
- 2 tablespoons olive oil
- 2 tablespoons lime juice
- 1 teaspoon ground cumin
- Salt and pepper to taste
- Avocado slices for serving
- Radish slices for garnish

Step-by-Step Instructions:

1. Cook quinoa according to package guidelines and let it cool.
2. In a large bowl, combine cooked quinoa, black beans, corn, diced red bell pepper, red onion, and cilantro.
3. In a small bowl, mix together olive oil, lime juice, ground cumin, salt, and pepper.
4. Pour the dressing over the quinoa mixture and toss gently.
5. Serve in bowls, topped with avocado slices and decorated with radish pieces.

Nutritional Information:

Calories: 320g | Protein: 12g | Fiber: 10g | Fats: 10g | Carbohydrates: 45g

Pro Tips:

- Add a bit of hot sauce for a spicy kick.
- Make a big batch and enjoy as a cool lunch the next day.

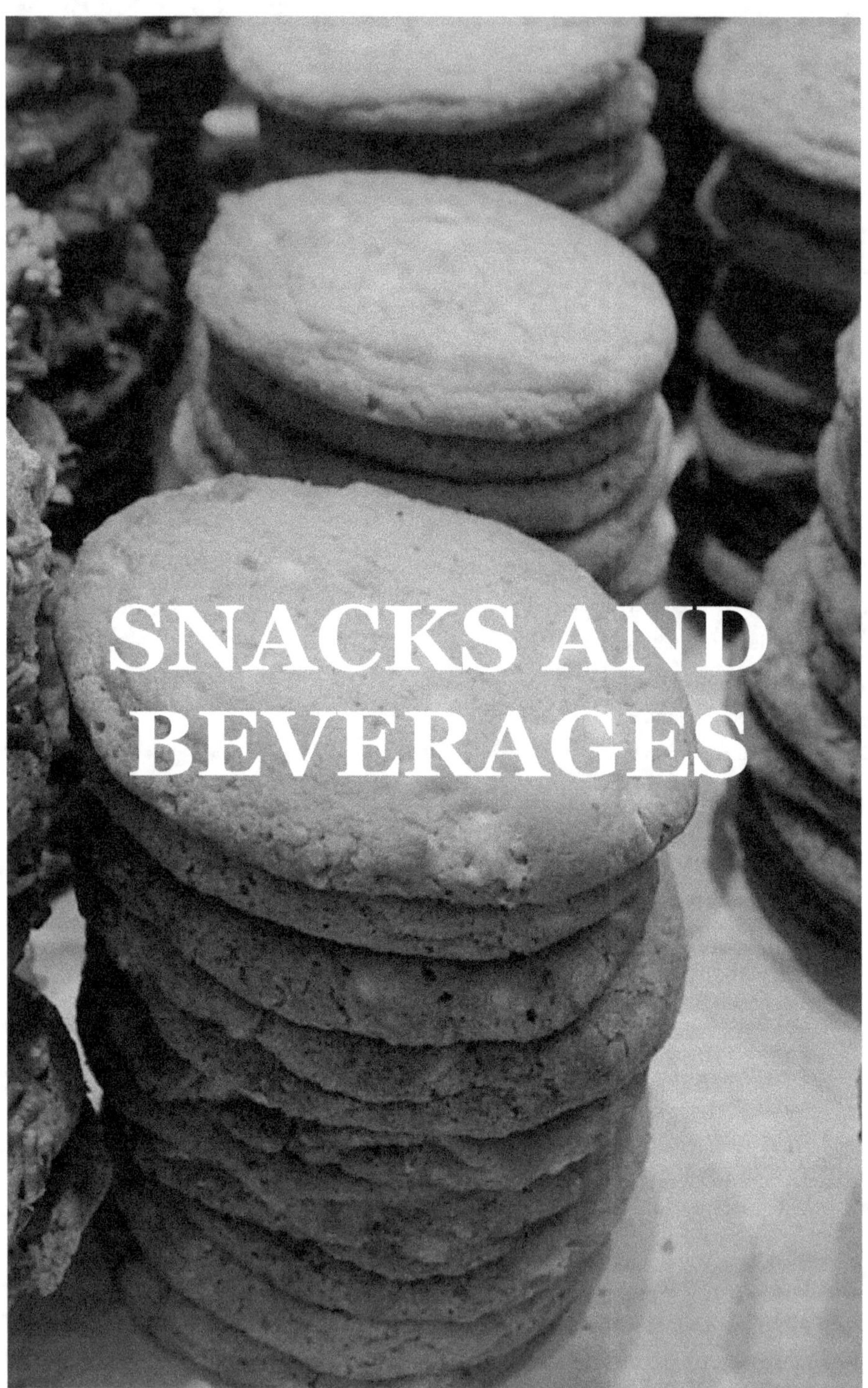

SNACKS AND BEVERAGES

Energize your day with our Almond Energy Bites. Packed with healthy ingredients like almonds, dates, and oats, these bites are a delicious and nutritious snack to keep you fed throughout the day.

Prep Time: 15 minutes
Cook Time: 30 minutes
Serves 12 bites

Ingredients:

- 1 cup almonds
- 1 cup chopped dates
- 1/2 cup rolled oats 2 tablespoons almond butter
- 1 tablespoon chia seeds
- 1 teaspoon vanilla flavor
- Pinch of salt
- Shredded coconut for coating (optional)

Step-by-Step Instructions:

1. In a food processor, blend almonds until finely chopped.
2. Add dates, oats, almond butter, chia seeds, vanilla extract, and a pinch of salt. Process until the mixture forms a sticky dough.
3. Scoop out tablespoon-sized pieces and roll into balls.
4. If wanted, roll the balls in shredded coconut for an extra layer of taste.
5. Allow to chill in the refrigerator for at least 30 minutes before serving.

Nutritional Information:

Calories: 90g | Protein: 3g | Fiber: 2g | Fats: 5g | Carbohydrates: 10g

Pro Tips:

- Customize with your favorite nuts or seeds.
- Store in a sealed jar in the fridge for a grab-and-go snack.

Nourish your body with our Herbal Infusions for Hormonal Balance. Sip on the goodness of plant teas made with ingredients known for their helpful effects on hormonal health.

Prep Time: 5 minutes
Cook Time: 10 minutes
Serves: 2 cups

Ingredients:
- 1 tablespoon dried chamomile flowers
- 1 tablespoon dried red clover flowers
- 1 tablespoon dried nettle leaves
- 2 cups hot water
- Honey or lemon (optional)

Step-by-Step Instructions:
1. In a teapot or heatproof pitcher, combine chamomile flowers, red clover blossoms, and nettle leaves.
2. Pour hot water over the herbs.
3. Allow the herbs to steep for 10 minutes.
4. Strain the mixture into cups.
5. Sweeten with honey or add a squeeze of lemon if wanted.

Pro Tips:
- Enjoy this herbal infusion daily for its potential hormonal balancing benefits.
- Experiment with other herbs like raspberry leaf or spearmint for variation.

Dip into freshness with our Guacamole and Veggie Sticks. Creamy avocado mixed with colorful veggies makes a filling and healthy snack that's great for any time of the day.

Prep Time: 15 minutes

Makes: 2 cups of guacamole

Ingredients:

- 3 ripe avocados, mashed 1 tomato, diced
- 1/4 cup red onion, finely chopped 1/4 cup fresh cilantro, chopped 1 clove garlic, minced
- Juice of 1 lime
- Salt and pepper to taste
- Assorted vegetable sticks (carrots, cucumber, bell peppers) for dipping

Step-by-Step Instructions:

1. In a bowl, mix mashed avocados, diced tomato, red onion, cilantro, chopped garlic, and lime juice.
2. Mix until well combined.
3. Season with salt and pepper to taste.
4. Serve with a variety of veggie sticks for dipping.

Pro Tips:

- Add a pinch of cayenne pepper for a hot kick.
- Store guacamole in a sealed container with a piece of plastic wrap put directly onto the top to avoid burning.

Indulge in a guilt-free treat with our Chocolate Avocado Mousse. Creamy avocados mixed with rich cocoa make a luscious and delicious mousse that fills your sweet needs.

Prep Time: 10 minutes

Cook Time: 2 hours

Serves: 4 serves

Ingredients:

- 2 ripe avocados
- 1/4 cup cocoa powder
- 1/4 cup maple syrup
- 1 teaspoon vanilla extract Pinch of salt
- Fresh berries for garnish

Step-by-Step Instructions:

1. Scoop the flesh of the avocados into a blender or food processor.
2. Add cocoa powder, maple syrup, vanilla extract, and a pinch of salt.
3. Blend until smooth and creamy.
4. Divide the mousse into serving cups.
5. Chill in the refrigerator for at least 2 hours.
6. Garnish with fresh berries before serving.

Nutritional Information:

Calories: 180g | Protein: 2g | Fiber: 6g | Fats: 12g | Carbohydrates: 20g

Pro Tips:

- Experiment with adding a dash of cinnamon or a shot of espresso for extra taste.
- Top with chopped nuts for extra crunch.

Start your day right or enjoy a healthy snack with our Berry and Chia Seed Pudding. Packed with chia seeds and a mix of berries, this pudding is a healthy and tasty treat.

Prep Time: 10 minutes

Cook Time: 4 hours or overnight

Serves: 2

Ingredients:
- 1/4 cup chia seeds
- 1 cup almond milk
- 1 tablespoon maple syrup
- 1/2 teaspoon vanilla extract
- 1 cup mixed berries (strawberries, blueberries, raspberries)
- Granola for topping (optional)

Step-by-Step Instructions:
1. In a bowl, mix together chia seeds, almond milk, maple syrup, and vanilla extract.
2. Let the mixture sit for 5 minutes, then whisk again to prevent clumps.
3. Cover the bowl and chill for at least 4 hours or overnight.
4. Before serving, give the pudding a good stir.
5. Layer the chia pudding with mixed berries and top with granola if desired.

Nutritional Information:
Calories: 180g | Protein: 4g | Fiber: 10g | Fats: 8g | Carbohydrates: 22g

Pro Tips:
- Customize with your favorite veggies or add a spoonful of yogurt.
- Make a batch for meal prep and enjoy throughout the week.

Satisfy your sweet tooth guilt-free with our Banana-Oat Cookies. These naturally sweetened cookies, made with ripe bananas and oats, are a delicious and healthy treat for any time of the day.

Prep Time: 15 minutes
Bake Time: 15 minutes
Makes: 12 cookies

Ingredients:

- 2 ripe bananas, mashed
- 1 cup rolled oats
- 1/4 cup almond butter
- 1/4 cup raisins or chocolate chips
- 1 teaspoon vanilla flavor
- 1/2 teaspoon cinnamon
- Pinch of salt

Step-by-Step Instructions:

1. Preheat the oven to 350°F (180°C) and prepare a baking sheet with parchment paper.
2. In a bowl, mix mashed bananas, rolled oats, almond butter, raisins or chocolate chips, vanilla extract, cinnamon, and a pinch of salt.
3. Mix until well mixed.
4. Drop spoonfuls of the batter onto the prepped baking sheet.
5. Bake for 15 minutes or until the sides are golden.
6. Allow to cool before eating.

Nutritional Information:

Calories: 80g | Protein: 2g | Fiber: 2g | Fats: 3g | Carbohydrates: 12g

Pro Tips:

- Experiment with adding nuts or seeds for extra crunch.
- Store in a sealed jar for freshness.

Refresh and revive with our Detoxifying Cucumber Gazpacho. This cool soup, featuring cucumbers, tomatoes, and herbs, is a refreshing and cleaning choice for a light and delicious snack.

Prep Time: 15 minutes

Chill Time: 1 hour

Makes: 4 serves

Ingredients:

- 2 peeled cucumbers and 4 large chopped tomatoes
- 1 Chopped red bell peppe
- ½ Chopped red onion
- Chopped 2 cloves garlic
- Minced 1/4 cup fresh basil
- Chopped 2 tablespoons fresh mint
- Chopped 3 cups vegetable broth
- 1/4 cup red wine vinegar
- Salt and pepper to taste
- Olive oil for drizzling
- Fresh herbs for garnish

Step-by-Step Instructions:

1. In a mixer, add cucumbers, tomatoes, red bell pepper, red onion, garlic, basil, mint, veggie broth, and red wine vinegar.
2. Blend until smooth.
3. Season with salt and pepper to taste.
4. Allow to chill in the refrigerator for at least 1 hour.
5. Before serving, spread with olive oil and top with fresh herbs.

Nutritional Information:

Calories: 60g | Protein: 2g | Fiber: 3g | Fats: 1g Carbohydrates: 12g

Pro Tips:

- Serve with a dash of black pepper for extra kick.
- Customize with your favorite herbs and spices.

Elevate your eating experience with our Spinach and Artichoke Dip. Creamy, cheesy, and full of flavor, this dip pairs perfectly with whole-grain crackers or veggie sticks for a wonderful treat.

Prep Time: 20 minutes
Bake Time: 25 minutes
Makes: 2 cups of dip

Ingredients:

- 1 cup frozen chopped spinach, thawed and drained
- 1 can (14 oz) artichoke hearts, drained and chopped
- 1 cup vegan cream cheese
- 1/2 cup vegan mayonnaise
- 1 cup vegan shredded mozzarella
- 1/2 cup healthy yeast
- 2 cloves garlic, minced
- 1 teaspoon onion powder
- Salt and pepper to taste
- Whole-grain bread or veggie sticks for dipping

Step-by-Step Instructions:

1. Preheat the oven to 375°F (190°C).
2. In a bowl, mix chopped spinach, chopped artichoke hearts, vegan cream cheese, vegan mayonnaise, vegan shredded mozzarella, nutritional yeast, minced garlic, onion powder, salt, and pepper.
3. Mix until well mixed.
4. Transfer the mixture to a baking dish.
5. Bake for 25 minutes or until the top is golden and bubbly.
6. Allow to cool slightly before serving with whole-grain bread or veggie sticks.

Pro Tips:

- Garnish with chopped fresh herbs for a burst of brightness.
- Double the recipe for a crowd-pleasing party dip.

HUMMUS-STUFFED BELL PEPPERS

Elevate your eating game with our Hummus-Stuffed Bell Peppers. These bright and crunchy pepper boats filled with creamy hummus make for a satisfying and nutritious snack.

Prep Time: 15 minutes
Makes: 8 stuffed pepper halves

Ingredients:

- 4 big bell peppers, split and seeds removed
- 1 cup hummus (store-bought or homemade)
- Cherry tomatoes, sliced, for garnish
- Fresh parsley, chopped, for garnish
- Olive oil for drizzling
- Crackers or pita bread for serving

Step-by-Step Instructions:

1. Fill each bell pepper half with a heaping spoonful of hummus.
2. Top with split cherry tomatoes and chopped fresh parsley.
3. Drizzle with olive oil before serving.
4. Arrange on a plate with crackers or pita bread.

Pro Tips:

- Choose a range of bell pepper colors for an eye-catching show.
- Sprinkle with a pinch of smoked paprika for extra taste.

Dive into the freshness of our Avocado and Black Bean Salsa. With creamy avocados, protein-packed black beans, and a spicy lime dressing, this salsa is a bright and filling snack.

Prep Time: 15 minutes
Makes: 3 cups of salsa

- **Ingredients:**
- 2 avocados, diced
- 1 can (15 oz) black beans, drained and washed
- 1 cup corn kernels (fresh or frozen)
- 1/2 red onion, roughly chopped
- 1 jalapeño, seeds and diced
- Juice of 2 limes
- 1/4 cup fresh cilantro, chopped
- Salt and pepper to taste
- Tortilla chips for dipping

Step-by-Step Instructions:
1. In a bowl, mix diced avocados, black beans, corn, red onion, jalapeño, lime juice, and chopped cilantro.
2. Gently toss until well mixed.
3. Season with salt and pepper to taste.
4. Serve with Mexican chips for dipping.

Pro Tips:
- Add a bit of chili pepper for extra heat.
- Refrigerate any extras in a sealed jar.

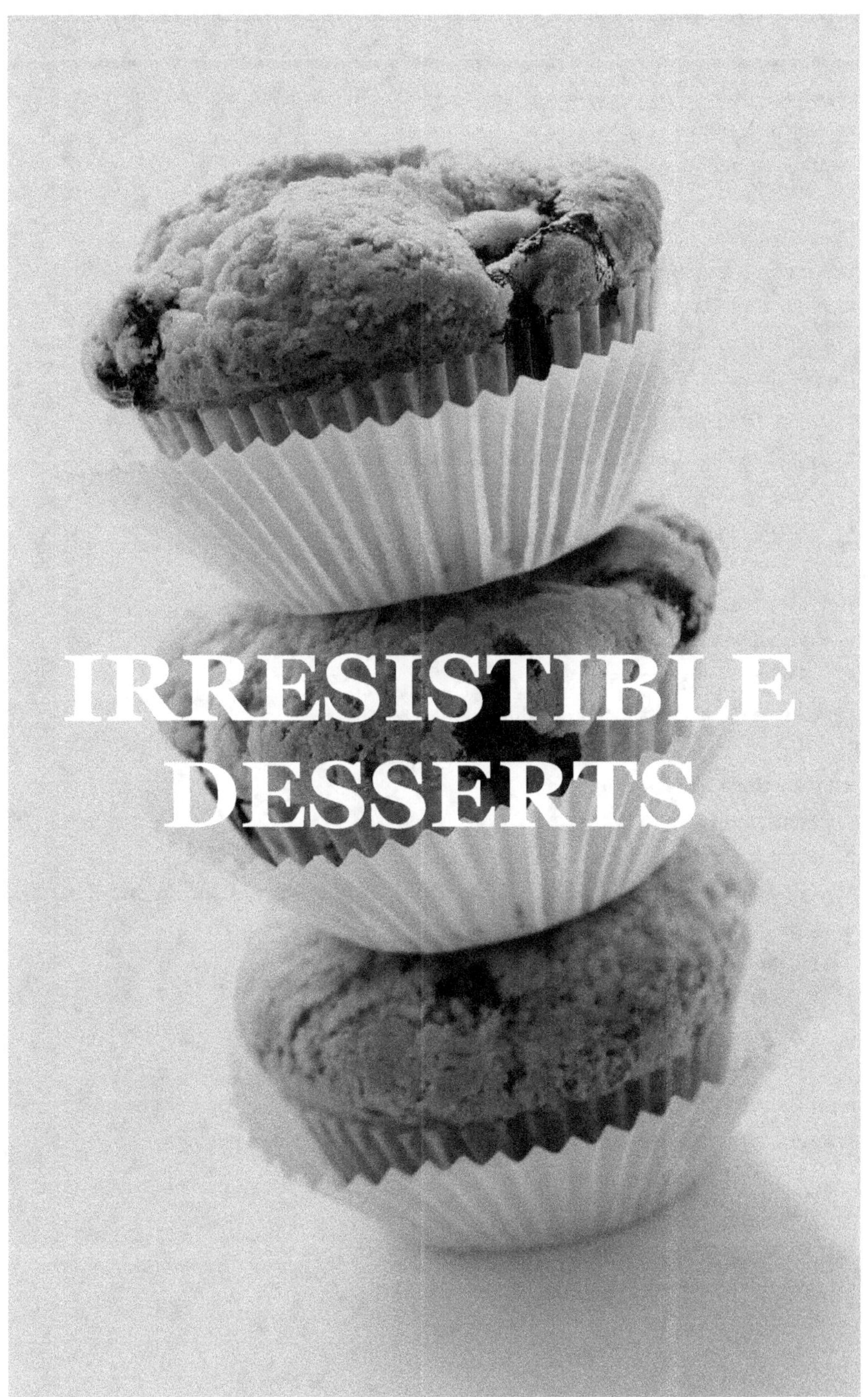

IRRESISTIBLE
DESSERTS

QUINOA-STUFFED ACORN SQUASH

Experience a burst of fall tastes with our Quinoa-Stuffed Acorn Squash. This hearty and healthy dish combines the nuttiness of quinoa with the sweetness of roasted acorn squash, creating a dinner that's as delicious as it is nutritious.

Prep Time: 20 minutes
Bake Time: 45 minutes
Serves: 4

Ingredients:

- 2 acorn squash, split and seeds removed
- 1 cup quinoa, cooked 1 can (15 oz) chickpeas, drained and washed
- 1/2 cup dried cranberries
- 1/2 cup pecans, chopped
- 1/4 cup fresh parsley, chopped
- 1 teaspoon ground cumin
- 1 teaspoon cinnamon
- Salt and pepper to taste
- Maple tahini dressing for drizzling

Step-by-Step Instructions:

1. Preheat the oven to 375°F (190°C).
2. Place acorn squash halves on a baking sheet, cut side up.
3. In a bowl, combine cooked quinoa, chickpeas, dried cranberries, pecans, fresh parsley, ground cumin, cinnamon, salt, and pepper.
4. Fill half of an acorn squash with the quinoa mixture.
5. Bake for 45 minutes, or until the squash is tender.
6. Drizzle with maple tahini dressing before serving.

Nutritional Information:

Calories: 380g | Protein: 10g | Fiber: 12g | Fats: 10g | Carbohydrates: 65g

Pro Tips:

- Experiment with different nuts or add a sprinkle of feta cheese.
- Serve with a side of sautéed greens for a full meal.

Elevate your dinner with our Lentil and Mushroom Stuffed Bell Peppers. Packed with protein-rich lentils, tasty mushrooms, and a mix of aromatic spices, these stuffed peppers are a flavorful and satisfying choice for a plant-powered meal.

Prep Time: 30 minutes

Bake Time: 30 minutes

Serves: 4

Ingredients:

- 4 big bell peppers, split and seeds removed
- 1 cup dry green lentils, cooked
- 1 cup mushrooms, finely chopped
- 1 onion, finely diced
- 2 cloves garlic, minced
- 1 teaspoon ground cumin
- 1 teaspoon smoked paprika
- 1/2 teaspoon chili powder
- Salt and pepper to taste
- 1 can (15 oz) chopped tomatoes
- 1 cup veggie broth
- Fresh cilantro for garnish

Step-by-Step Instructions:

1. Preheat the oven to 375°F (190°C).
2. In a pan, sauté mushrooms, onion, and garlic until cooked.
3. Add cooked lentils, ground cumin, smoked paprika, chili powder, salt, and pepper. Stir well.
4. Pour in chopped tomatoes and veggie stock. Simmer until the liquid is absorbed.
5. Fill each bell pepper half with the lentil and mushroom mixture.
6. Bake for 30 minutes or until peppers are soft.
7. Garnish with fresh cilantro before serving.

Nutritional Information:

Calories: 320g | Protein: 15g | Fiber: 12g | Fats: 5g | Carbohydrates: 50g

Pro Tips:

- Top with a spoonful of vegan sour cream or yogurt.

Transport your taste buds to the tropics with our Coconut Curry Chickpea Bowl. This aromatic and creamy curry, featuring chickpeas, vegetables, and coconut milk, is a delightful and comforting choice for a flavorful dinner.

Prep Time: 25 minutes

Cook Time: 30 minutes

Serves: 4

Ingredients:

- 1 can (15 oz) chickpeas, drained and washed
- 1 sweet potato, diced
- 1 cup cauliflower sprouts
- 1 cup broccoli stems
- 1 bell pepper, sliced
- 1 onion, finely chopped
- 2 cloves garlic, minced
- 1 can (14 oz) coconut milk
- 2 tablespoons red curry paste
- 1 tablespoon soy sauce
- 1 tablespoon maple syrup
- Juice of 1 lime
- Cooked brown rice for serving
- Fresh cilantro for garnish

Step-by-Step Instructions:

1. In a pan, sauté onion and garlic until fragrant.
2. Add sweet potato, cauliflower, broccoli, and bell pepper. Cook until slightly softened.
3. Stir in chickpeas, coconut milk, red curry paste, soy sauce, maple syrup, and lime juice.
4. Simmer until veggies are soft and the curry thickens.
5. Serve over cooked brown rice and top with fresh cilantro.

Nutritional Information:

Calories: 420g | Protein: 12g | Fiber: 10g | Fats: 20g | Carbohydrates: 55g

Pro Tips:

- Customize with your favorite veggies or add tofu for extra nutrition.
- Adjust the level of spice by varying the amount of red curry paste.

Indulge in the rich and creamy tastes of our Chickpea and Spinach Coconut Curry. With a medley of spices, chickpeas, and nutrient-packed spinach, this curry is a quick and satisfying option for a delicious dinner.

Prep Time: 15 minutes

Cook Time: 25 minutes

Serves: 4

Ingredients:

- 1 can (15 oz) chickpeas, drained and washed
- 1 onion, finely chopped
- 2 cloves garlic, minced
- 1 teaspoon ground cumin 1 teaspoon ground coriander
- 1 teaspoon turmeric
- 1/2 teaspoon chili pepper
- 1 can (14 oz) coconut milk
- 1 can (14 oz) diced tomatoes
- 4 cups fresh spinach
- Salt and pepper to taste
- Cooked basmati rice for serving
- Fresh cilantro for garnish

Step-by-Step Instructions:

1. In a pan, sauté onion and garlic until cooked.
2. Add ground cumin, ground coriander, turmeric, and cayenne pepper. Stir well.
3. Pour in coconut milk and diced tomatoes. Simmer for 10 minutes.
4. Add chickpeas and fresh spinach. Cook until spinach wilts.
5. Season with salt and pepper to taste.
6. Serve with cooked basmati rice and fresh cilantro on top.

Nutritional Information:

Calories: 380g | Protein: 14g | Fiber: 10g | Fats: 15g | Carbohydrates: 50g

Pro Tips:

- Customize the spice amount to fit your taste.
- Add a squeeze of fresh lemon or lime juice before serving.

Embrace the freshness of our Zucchini Noodles with Pesto. This light and tasty dish feature spiralized zucchini noodles tossed in a bright basil pesto, creating a low-carb and nutrient-packed dinner that's as filling as it is delicious.

Prep Time: 15 minutes
Cook Time: 5 minutes
Serves: 2

Ingredients:
- 4 medium zucchinis, spiralized
- 1 cup cherry tomatoes, sliced
- 1/2 cup pine nuts, toasted
- 1/2 cup fresh basil leaves
- 1/4 cup healthy yeast
- 2 cloves garlic
- Juice of 1 lemon
- 1/2 cup extra-virgin olive oil
- Salt and pepper to taste
- Vegan Parmesan for garnish

Step-by-Step Instructions:
1. In a mixer or food processor, add fresh basil, pine nuts, nutritional yeast, garlic, and lemon juice.
2. With the blender going, slowly pour in the olive oil until the pesto is smooth.
3. In a pan, quickly sauté spiralized zucchini noodles until just tender.
4. Toss the zucchini noodles with the cherry tomatoes and pesto.
5. Season with salt and pepper to taste.
6. Garnish with veggie Parmesan before serving.

Nutritional Information:
Calories: 320g | Protein: 8g | Fiber: 6g | Fats: 28g | Carbohydrates: 12g

Pro Tips:
- Top with extra toasted pine nuts for crunch.
- Add grilled tofu or chickpeas for extra nutrition.

Delight your taste buds with our Stuffed Bell Peppers featuring protein-packed quinoa. These colorful peppers are filled with a savory mixture of quinoa, black beans, corn, and spices, creating a wholesome and satisfying dinner.

Prep Time: 20 minutes

Bake Time: 30 minutes

Serves: 4

Ingredients:

- 4 big bell peppers, split and seeds removed
- 1 cup quinoa, cooked
- 1 can (15 oz) black beans, drained and washed
- 1 cup corn kernels (fresh or frozen)
- 1 onion, finely chopped
- 2 cloves garlic, minced
- 1 teaspoon crushed cumin
- 1 teaspoon chili powder
- Salt and pepper to taste
- 1 cup tomato sauce
- Vegan cheese for topping (optional)

Step-by-Step Instructions:

1. Preheat the oven to 375°F (190°C).
2. In a pan, sauté onion and garlic until cooked.
3. Add cooked quinoa, black beans, corn, ground cumin, chili powder, salt, and pepper. Mix well.
4. Fill each bell pepper half with the rice filling.
5. Pour tomato sauce over the stuffed peppers.
6. Bake for 30 minutes or until peppers are soft.
7. If wanted, sprinkle with vegan cheese and bake until melted.

Nutritional Information:

Calories: 340g | Protein: 12g | Fiber: 10g | Fats: 5g | Carbohydrates: 60g

Pro Tips:

- Customize with your favorite toppings like avocado or salsa.

PLANT-BASED STIR-FRY

Embark on a culinary journey with our Plant-Based Stir-Fry, a vibrant medley of colorful vegetables and tofu, wok-tossed in a savory and umami-rich sauce. This quick and tasty stir-fry is great for a healthy dinner.

Prep Time: 15 minutes

Cook Time: 10 minutes

Serves: 4

Ingredients:

- 1 block firm tofu, pressed and cubed
- 2 cups broccoli florets
- 1 bell pepper, sliced
- 1 carrot, julienned
- 1 cup snap peas
- 1/2 cup baby corn
- 3 cloves garlic, minced
- 1 tablespoon ginger, grated
- 1/4 cup soy sauce
- 2 tablespoons hoisin sauce
- 1 tablespoon sesame oil
- Cooked brown rice for serving
- Green onions for garnish

Step-by-Step Instructions:

1. In a wok or big pan, sauté tofu cubes until golden brown. Set aside.
2. In the same pan, stir-fry broccoli, bell pepper, carrot, snap peas, and baby corn until crisp-tender.
3. Add chopped garlic and grated ginger. Stir-fry for an extra minute.
4. Return the tofu to the pan.
5. In a small bowl, mix together soy sauce, hoisin sauce, and sesame oil. Pour over the stir-fry.
6. Toss everything until well coated and heated through.
7. Serve over cooked brown rice and garnish with green onions.

Nutritional Information:

Calories: 320g | Protein: 15g | Fiber: 8g | Fats: 10g | Carbohydrates: 45g

Pro Tips:

- For added crunch, sprinkle with sesame seeds.

Warm your heart with a bowl of our hearty Minestrone Soup. This hearty and healthy soup features a mix of veggies, beans, and pasta, cooked to perfection in a delicious tomato broth. A great choice for a comforting and filling dinner.

Prep Time: 20 minutes

Cook Time: 30 minutes

Serves: 6

Ingredients:

- 1 tablespoon olive oil
- 1 onion, finely chopped
- 2 carrots, diced
- 2 celery stalks, diced
- 3 cloves garlic, minced 1 can (15 oz) kidney beans, washed and rinsed
- 1 can (15 oz) diced tomatoes
- 6 cups vegetable broth 1 cup small pasta (e.g., ditalini or elbow)
- 2 teaspoons Italian seasoning
- Salt and pepper to taste
- 2 cups fresh spinach, chopped
- Fresh basil for garnish
- Vegan Parmesan for serving

Step-by-Step Instructions:

1. In a big pot, heat olive oil over medium heat.
2. Sauté onion, carrots, celery, and garlic until softened.
3. Add kidney beans, chopped tomatoes, veggie broth, pasta, Italian spice, salt, and pepper. Simmer until pasta is cooked.
4. Stir in chopped spinach and cook until softened.
5. Garnish with fresh basil and serve with vegan Parmesan.

Nutritional Information:

Calories: 250g | Protein: 10g | Fiber: 8g | Fats: 5g | Carbohydrates: 40g

Pro Tips:

- Customize with your favorite veggies or add cannellini beans.
- Make a big batch for leftovers—it tastes even better the next day!

Elevate your dinner with our Quinoa and Black Bean Salad, a delicious and protein-packed dish that blends quinoa, black beans, fresh veggies, and a zesty lime dressing. This salad is great for a light and healthy meal.

Prep Time: 15 minutes
Serves: 4

Ingredients:

- 1 cup quinoa, cooked and cooled
- 1 can (15 oz) black beans, drained and washed
- 1 cup corn kernels (fresh or frozen), cooked
- 1 red bell pepper, diced
- 1/2 red onion, finely chopped
- 1/4 cup fresh cilantro, chopped
- Juice of 2 limes
- 2 tablespoons olive oil
- 1 teaspoon cumin
- Salt and pepper to taste
- Avocado slices for garnish

Step-by-Step Instructions:

1. In a large bowl, combine cooked quinoa, black beans, corn, red bell pepper, red onion, and cilantro.
2. In a small bowl, mix together lime juice, olive oil, cumin, salt, and pepper.
3. Pour the dressing over the salad and toss until well mixed.
4. Garnish with avocado slices before serving.

Nutritional Information:

Calories: 320 | Protein: 12g | Fiber: 10g | Fats: 10g | Carbohydrates: 50g

Pro Tips:

- Add a touch of chili powder for a bit of spice.
- Serve cold for a relaxing experience.

DETOXIFYING CUCUMBER GAZPACHO

Revitalize your senses with our Detoxifying Cucumber Gazpacho—a refreshing and hydrating soup that mixes the crispness of cucumbers with the brightness of tomatoes and herbs. This gazpacho is great for a light and filling dinner.

Prep Time: 15 minutes

Chill Time: 1 hour

Serves: 4

Ingredients:

- 4 large cucumbers, peeled and chopped
- 4 large tomatoes, chopped 1 red bell pepper, chopped 1/2 red onion, chopped 2 cloves garlic, minced 1/4 cup fresh basil, chopped 2 tablespoons fresh mint, chopped 3 cups vegetable broth
- 1/4 cup red wine vinegar
- Salt and pepper to taste
- Olive oil for drizzling
- Fresh herbs for garnish

Step-by-Step Instructions:

1. In a mixer, add cucumbers, tomatoes, red bell pepper, red onion, garlic, basil, mint, veggie broth, and red wine vinegar.
2. Blend until smooth.
3. Season with salt and pepper to taste.
4. Allow to chill in the refrigerator for at least 1 hour.
5. Before serving, drizzle with olive oil and garnish with fresh herbs.

Nutritional Information:

Calories: 60 | Protein: 2g | Fiber: 3g | Fats: 1g | Carbohydrates: 12g

Pro Tips:

- Serve with a sprinkle of black pepper for added kick.
- Customize with your favorite herbs and spices.

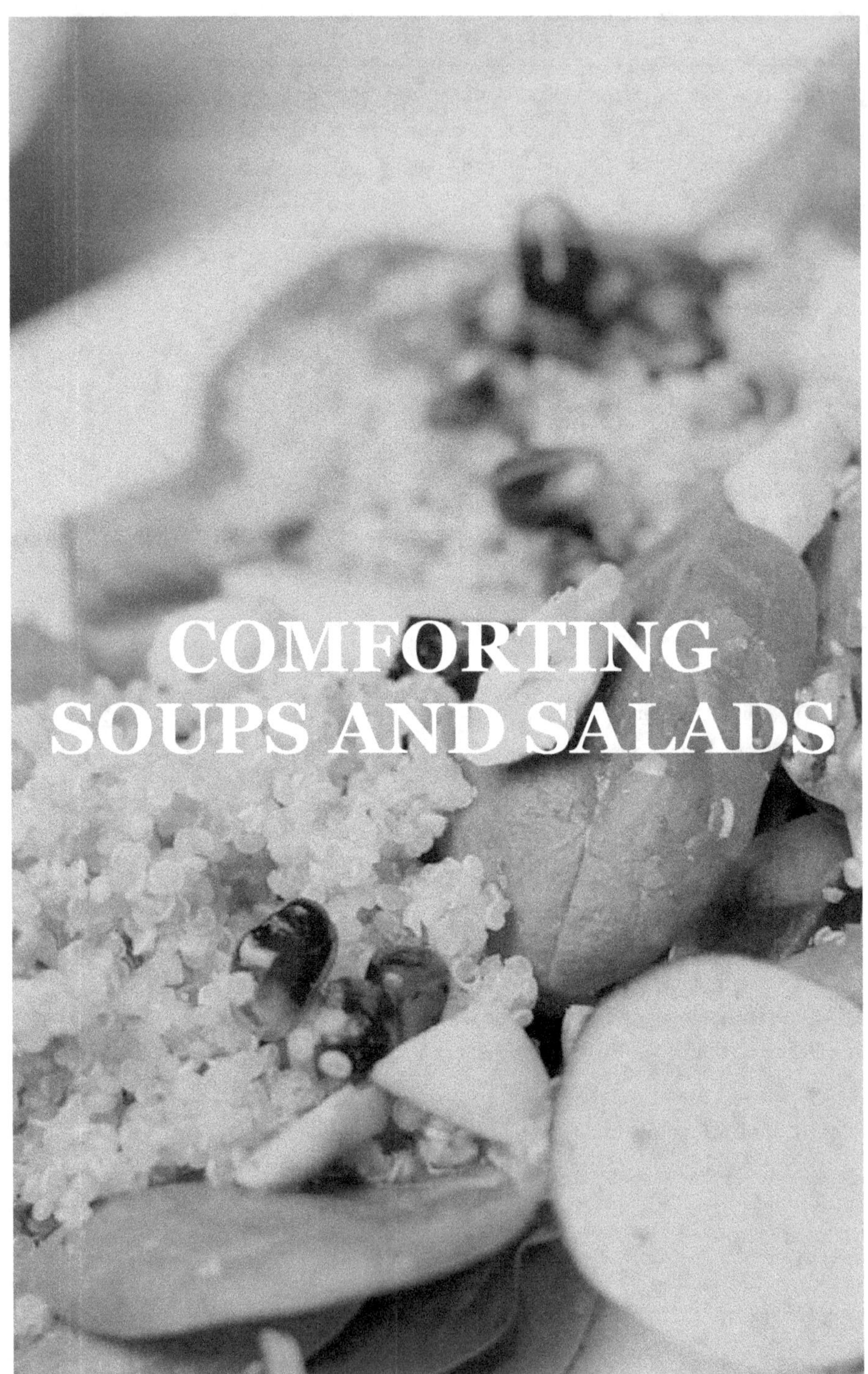

COMFORTING SOUPS AND SALADS

Warm up with our Hearty Lentil and Vegetable Soup—a comforting mix of protein-rich lentils, bright veggies, and savory herbs. This filling soup is great for a cozy and delicious dinner.

Prep Time: 15 minutes
Cook Time: 35 minutes
Serves: 6

Ingredients:

- 1 cup dry green lentils, rinsed
- 1 onion, finely chopped 2 carrots, diced 2 celery stalks, diced 3 cloves garlic, minced 1 can (15 oz) diced tomatoes
- 6 cups vegetable broth
- 1 teaspoon crushed cumin
- 1 teaspoon smoked paprika
- 1/2 teaspoon thyme
- Salt and pepper to taste
- Fresh parsley for garnish

Step-by-Step Instructions:

1. In a big pot, sauté onion, carrots, celery, and garlic until softened.
2. Add lentils, diced tomatoes, veggie broth, ground cumin, smoked paprika, thyme, salt, and pepper. Simmer until lentils are tender.
3. Adjust seasoning to taste.
4. Garnish with fresh parsley before serving.

Nutritional Information:

Calories: 280g | Protein: 15g | Fiber: 8g | Fats: 3g | Carbohydrates: 45g

Pro Tips:

- Serve with a slice of fresh whole-grain bread.
- Make a large batch for quick meal preparation.

Transport your taste buds to Thailand with our Thai-Inspired Coconut Curry Soup. This aromatic and creamy soup features coconut milk, red curry paste, and a variety of veggies, creating a balanced blend of flavors perfect for a delightful dinner.

Prep Time: 20 minutes

Cook Time: 25 minutes

Serves: 4

Ingredients:

- 1 tablespoon coconut oil
- 1 onion, finely chopped
- 2 carrots, julienned 1 red bell pepper, sliced
- 3 cloves garlic, minced
- 2 tablespoons red curry paste
- 1 can (14 oz) coconut milk
- 4 cups vegetable broth
- 1 tablespoon soy sauce
- 1 tablespoon maple syrup
- Juice of 1 lime
- Rice noodles for serving
- Fresh cilantro for garnish

Step-by-Step Instructions:

1. In a pot, heat coconut oil over medium heat.
2. Sauté onion, carrots, red bell pepper, and garlic until softened.
3. Add red curry paste and stir well.
4. Pour in coconut milk, veggie broth, soy sauce, maple syrup, and lime juice. Simmer for 15 minutes.
5. Cook rice noodles according to package directions.
6. Serve the soup over rice noodles and top with fresh cilantro.

Nutritional Information:

Calories: 32g | Protein: 8g | Fiber: 6g |Fats: 15g | Carbohydrates: 40g

Pro Tips:

- Customize with your favorite veggies or add tofu.
- Adjust the spice level by varying the amount of red curry paste.

Elevate your dinner with our Mediterranean Chickpea Salad—a bright and protein-packed dish that blends chickpeas, colored veggies, and a zesty lemon dressing. This refreshing salad is great for a light and healthy meal.

Prep Time: 15 minutes
Serves: 4

Ingredients:

- 2 cans (15 oz each) chickpeas
- 1 Drained and rinsed cucumber
- 1 Diced cup cherry tomatoes
- 1 Halved red onion
- 1/2 cup of Finely chopped Kalamata olives
- ½ cup of Sliced fresh parsley
- ¼ cup of Chopped 1/4 extra-virgin olive oil
- Juice of 2 lemons
- 1 teaspoon dried oregano
- Salt and pepper to taste
- Feta cheese for garnish (optional)

Step-by-Step Instructions:

1. In a large bowl, combine chickpeas, cucumber, cherry tomatoes, red onion, Kalamata olives, and fresh parsley.
2. In a small bowl, mix together olive oil, lemon juice, dried oregano, salt, and pepper.
3. Toss the salad with the dressing until completely combined.
4. Garnish with chopped feta cheese if wanted.

Nutritional Information:

Calories: 320g | Protein: 12g | Fiber: 10g | Fats: 15g | Carbohydrates: 40g

Pro Tips:

- Serve with whole-grain pita bread for a full meal.
- Make it ahead for a quick and filling lunch.

Introduction:

Savor the healthy goodness of our Quinoa and Black Bean Soup—a protein-packed treat featuring quinoa, black beans, veggies, and delicious spices. This filling soup is great for a rich and satisfying dinner.

Prep Time: 15 minutes

Cook Time: 25 minutes

Serves: 6

Ingredients:

- 1 cup quinoa, rinsed
- 1 can (15 oz) black beans, drained and washed
- 1 onion, finely chopped
- 2 carrots, diced 2 celery stalks, diced 3 cloves garlic, minced
- 1 can (15 oz) diced tomatoes
- 6 cups veggie broth 1 teaspoon cumin 1 teaspoon chili powder
- 1/2 teaspoon smoked paprika
- Salt and pepper to taste
- Avocado slices for garnish

Step-by-Step Instructions:

1. In a pot, sauté onion, carrots, celery, and garlic until cooked.
2. Add quinoa, black beans, diced tomatoes, vegetable broth, cumin, chili powder, smoked paprika, salt, and pepper. Simmer until quinoa is cooked.
3. Adjust seasoning to taste.
4. Garnish with avocado slices before serving.

Nutritional Information:

Calories: 290g | Protein: 12g | Fiber: 8g | Fats: 3g | Carbohydrates: 50g

Pro Tips:

- Top with a spoonful of vegan sour cream or yogurt.
- Add a splash of lime juice for extra zing.

Revitalize your taste with our Detox Salad featuring a bright spread of nutrient-packed veggies and a zesty lemon-tahini dressing. This crisp and crunchy salad is great for a light and healthy dinner.

Prep Time: 20 minutes

Serves: 4

Ingredients:

- 4 cups mixed greens (kale, spinach
- , arugula)
- 1 cup purple cabbage, shredded
- 1 carrot, julienned
- 1 beet, grated 1 cucumber, sliced
- 1 avocado, diced
- 1/4 cup pumpkin seeds
- 1/4 cup sunflower seeds
- 1/4 cup fresh cilantro, chopped
- Juice of 1 lemon
- 2 tablespoons tahini
- 1 tablespoon maple sugar
- Salt and pepper to taste

Step-by-Step Instructions:

1. In a big bowl, add mixed leaves, purple cabbage, carrot, beet, cucumber, avocado, pumpkin seeds, sunflower seeds, and cilantro.
2. In a small bowl, mix together lemon juice, tahini, maple syrup, salt, and pepper.
3. Pour the dressing over the salad and toss until well covered.
4. Serve quickly for best taste.

Nutritional Information:

Calories: 280g | Protein: 8g | Fiber: 10g | Fats: 18g | Carbohydrates: 30g

Pro Tips:

- Add grilled tofu or chickpeas for extra nutrition.
- Make a double amount of the dressing for future salads.

Indulge in the warmth and flavor of our Roasted Butternut Squash Soup. This creamy soup combines the sweet flavor of roasted butternut squash with aromatic spices, creating a warm and soul-soothing dinner choice.

Prep Time: 15 minutes

Roast Time: 40 minutes

Cook Time: 20 minutes

Serves: 4

Ingredients:

- 1 big butternut squash, peeled and diced
- 1 onion, chopped 2 carrots, chopped 3 cloves garlic, minced
- 1 teaspoon cumin
- 1/2 teaspoon cinnamon
- 1/4 teaspoon nutmeg
- 4 cups vegetable broth
- 1 cup coconut milk
- Salt and pepper to taste
- Pumpkin seeds for garnish

Step-by-Step Instructions:

1. Preheat the oven to 400°F (200°C).
2. Toss butternut squash, onion, carrots, and garlic with cumin, cinnamon, and nutmeg.
3. Roast for 40 minutes or until veggies are soft.
4. Transfer cooked veggies to a pot, add vegetable stock and coconut milk. Simmer for 20 minutes.
5. Blend until smooth using a hand blender.
6. Season with salt and pepper.
7. Garnish with pumpkin seeds before serving.

Nutritional Information:

Calories: 280g | Protein: 5g | Fiber: 8g | Fats: 10g | Carbohydrates: 40g

Pro Tips:

- Drizzle with a splash of coconut milk for an extra touch of sweetness.
- Serve with fresh whole-grain bread.

Delight your taste with our Spinach and Strawberry Salad—a delicious mix of bright spinach leaves, juicy strawberries, and crunchy almonds, all dressed in a light balsamic dressing. This salad is a great addition to your dinner table.

Prep Time: 10 minutes

Serves: 4

Ingredients:

- 6 cups fresh baby spinach
- 1 cup strawberries, hulled and sliced
- 1/2 cup sliced almonds, toasted 1/4 cup red onion, thinly sliced
- 1/4 cup feta cheese, crumbled
- Balsamic vinaigrette dressing

Step-by-Step Instructions:

1. In a big bowl, mix baby spinach, sliced strawberries, toasted almonds, red onion, and crumbled feta cheese.
2. Drizzle with balsamic vinaigrette dressing.
3. Toss gently until well coated.
4. Serve immediately to preserve the freshness.

Nutritional Information:

Calories: 180g | Protein: 6g | Fiber: 5g | Fats: 12g | Carbohydrates: 15g

Pro Tips:

- Add grilled chicken or tofu for a nutritional boost.
- Customize with your favorite nuts or seeds.

Nourish your body with our healthy Lentil and Vegetable Stew—a rich mix of lentils, various veggies, and flavorful herbs. This comforting stew is filled with flavor and makes for a satisfying and healthy dinner.

Prep Time: 15 minutes
Cook Time: 30 minutes
Serves: 6

Ingredients:

- 1 cup dry brown lentils, rinsed
- 1 onion, finely chopped 2 carrots, diced 2 celery stalks, diced 3 cloves garlic, minced 1 can (15 oz) diced tomatoes
- 6 cups vegetable broth
- 1 teaspoon dried thyme
- 1 teaspoon smoked paprika
- Salt and pepper to taste
- Fresh parsley for garnish

Step-by-Step Instructions:

1. In a pot, sauté onion, carrots, celery, and garlic until cooked.
2. Add brown lentils, diced tomatoes, veggie broth, thyme, smoked paprika, salt, and pepper. Simmer until lentils are tender.
3. Adjust seasoning to taste.
4. Garnish with fresh parsley before serving.

Nutritional Information:

Calories: 250g | Protein: 14g | Fiber: 8g | Fats: 2g | Carbohydrates: 45g

Pro Tips:

- Serve over cooked quinoa or brown rice.
- Make extra for a week of filling lunches.

CHICKPEA AND AVOCADO SALAD

Experience the wonderful balance of our Chickpea and Avocado Salad—a protein-packed combination featuring chickpeas, creamy avocado, cherry tomatoes, and a spicy lime sauce. This refreshing salad is a great addition to your dinner spread.

Prep Time: 15 minutes

Serves: 4

Ingredients:

- 2 cans (15 oz each) chickpeas, drained and washed
- 2 avocados, diced 1 cup cherry tomatoes, halved 1/4 cup red onion, finely chopped
- 1/4 cup fresh cilantro, chopped Juice of 2 limes
- 2 tablespoons olive oil
- Salt and pepper to taste

Step-by-Step Instructions:

1. In a big bowl, mix beans, diced avocados, cherry tomatoes, red onion, and fresh cilantro.
2. In a small bowl, mix together lime juice, olive oil, salt, and pepper.
3. Pour the dressing over the salad and toss gently until well mixed.
4. Serve quickly to enjoy the smooth taste.

Nutritional Information:

Calories: 320g | Protein: 12g | Fiber: 10g | Fats: 18g | Carbohydrates: 35g

Pro Tips:

- Add a dash of chili flakes for a touch of heat.
- Pair with grilled shrimp or tofu for extra energy.

Elevate your dinner with our Quinoa and Kale Salad—a nutrient-packed combination of quinoa, vibrant kale, roasted sweet potatoes, and a tangy tahini dressing. This healthy salad is both filling and nutritious.

Prep Time: 20 minutes
Cook Time: 25 minutes
Serves: 4

Ingredients:

- 1 cup quinoa, cooked and cooled
- 4 cups kale, destemmed and chopped
- 2 sweet potatoes, peeled and diced
- 1 tablespoon olive oil
- 1 teaspoon smoked paprika
- Salt and pepper to taste
- 1/4 cup pumpkin seeds, toasted
- 1/4 cup dried cranberries
- 1/4 cup feta cheese, crumbled Tahini dressing

Step-by-Step Instructions:

1. Preheat the oven to 400°F (200°C).
2. Toss sweet potatoes with olive oil, smoked paprika, salt, and pepper. Roast until tender.
3. In a big bowl, mix cooked quinoa, chopped kale, roasted sweet potatoes, pumpkin seeds, dried cranberries, and crumbled feta cheese.
4. Drizzle with tahini dressing and toss until well coated.
5. Serve quickly for a delicious dinner.

Nutritional Information:

Calories: 350g | Protein: 10g | Fiber: 8g | Fats: 12g | Carbohydrates: 55g

Pro Tips:

- Massage kale with a bit of olive oil for a tender texture.
- Customize with your favorite roasted veggies.

CONCLUSION

In closing the chapters of this Plant-Based PCOS Diet Cookbook, we find ourselves at the intersection of nourishment and empowerment. What began as a journey through the intricacies of PCOS and the labyrinth of health has transformed into a tapestry of vibrant recipes, insightful knowledge, and a renewed sense of well-being.

As you've navigated these pages, you've not only embraced the flavors of plant-based living but also embarked on a profound exploration of self-care. The recipes within these covers are not just culinary creations; they are a manifestation of the commitment to your health, your hormones, and your overall vitality.

From the energizing Green Smoothie Bowl to the comforting Detoxifying Cucumber Gazpacho, each recipe carries with it the intention to fuel your body with the richness of plant-based goodness. Together, they create a symphony of flavors that dance in harmony with your health goals, offering not just sustenance but an invitation to a more balanced and empowered life.

This cookbook is not just a collection of recipes; it's a catalyst for change. It's an invitation to embrace a lifestyle that transcends conventional norms, a shift towards a plant-powered existence that goes beyond the plate and permeates every aspect of your well-being.

As you take the last bite of a delectable plant-based creation, remember that this is not the end; it's a continuation of your journey. The knowledge gained, the recipes savored, and the holistic approach embraced are tools you carry forward.

Empowerment is not confined to the pages of this book; it's a gift you carry within. Your choices, your commitment to well-being, and your journey towards a healthier you are the true ingredients of this transformative experience.
Thank you for allowing me to be a part of your wellness journey. May these recipes continue to nourish not just your body but your spirit, fostering a life rich in vitality, balance, and the joy that comes from embracing your health wholeheartedly.

"Here's to the vibrant, empowered, and balanced you—today, tomorrow, and always."

	BREAKFAST	SNACK	LUNCH	DINNER
SUNDAY	Avocado Toast Variations	Almond Energy Bites	Chickpea and Spinach Salad	Stuffed Portobello Mushrooms
MONDAY	Quinoa and Berry Parfait	Herbal Infusions for Hormonal Balance	Lentil and Vegetable Wrap	Chickpea and Spinach Curry
TUESDAY	Green Smoothie Bowl	Guacamole and Veggie Sticks	Minestrone Soup	Plant-Based Stir-Fry
WEDNEDAY	Chickpea and Spinach Salad	Chocolate Avocado Mousse	Quinoa and Black Bean Soup	Spaghetti with Lentil Bolognese
THURSDAY	Lentil and Vegetable Wrap	Berry and Chia Seed Pudding	Detoxifying Cucumber Gazpacho	Zucchini Noodles with Tomato Sauce
FRIDAY	Sweet Potato and Kale Bowl	Banana-Oat Cookies	Mediterranean Chickpea Salad	Vegan Stuffed Bell Peppers
SATURDAY	Zucchini Noodles with Tomato Sauce	Minestrone Soup	Sweet Potato and Chickpea Buddha Bowl	Quinoa and Black Bean Salad

PRODUCE:

Avocado (4)

Berries (assorted, 1 pack)

Spinach (2 bunches)

Portobello Mushrooms (1 pack)

Quinoa (1 pack)

Fresh Herbs (assorted, 1 bunch)

Zucchini (3)

Tomato (4)

Sweet Potato (2)

Bell Peppers (assorted, 4)

Cherry Tomatoes (1 pack)

Red Onion (2)

Cucumber (2)

Kale (1 bunch)

Lemon (2)

Lime (2)

Strawberries (1 pack)

Fresh Cilantro (1 bunch)

Fresh Mint (1 bunch)

Garlic (1 pack)

PROTEINS:

Chickpeas (2 cans)

Lentils (1 pack)

Tofu (1 pack)

GRAINS:

Whole Wheat Wraps (1 pack)

DAIRY AND ALTERNATIVES:

Feta Cheese (1 pack)

Almond Butter (1 jar)

Coconut Milk (2 cans)

BAKERY:

Whole-Grain Bread (1 loaf)

NUTS AND SEEDS:

Almonds (1 pack)

Chia Seeds (1 pack)

Pumpkin Seeds (1 pack)

Sunflower Seeds (1 pack)

PANTRY STAPLES:

Olive Oil

Coconut Oil

Cumin

Cinnamon

Nutmeg

Red Curry Paste

Vegetable Broth (2 cartons)

Diced Tomatoes (2 cans)

Spaghetti (1 pack)

Tahini (1 jar)

Maple Syrup (1 bottle)

Black Beans (2 cans)

Quinoa and Black Bean Salad Ingredients

Brown Lentils

Smoked Paprika

Balsamic Vinaigrette Dressing

Lentil Bolognese Ingredients

Hummus (1 container)

BEVERAGES:

Herbal Infusions (assorted, 1 box)

	BREAKFAST	SNACK	LUNCH	DINNER
SUNDAY	Chickpea and Spinach Salad	Chocolate Avocado Mousse	Mediterranean Quinoa Bowl	Stuffed Bell Peppers with Quinoa
MONDAY	Quinoa and Black Bean Salad	Banana-Oat Cookies	Lentil and Vegetable Wrap	Vegan Stuffed Bell Peppers
TUESDAY	Avocado Toast Variations	Detoxifying Cucumber Gazpacho	Quinoa and Berry Parfait	Zucchini Noodles with Tomato Sauce
WEDNEDAY	Sweet Potato and Kale Bowl	Almond Energy Bites	Chickpea and Spinach Curry	Plant-Based Stir-Fry
THURSDAY	Green Smoothie Bowl	Guacamole and Veggie Sticks	Minestrone Soup	Spaghetti with Lentil Bolognese
FRIDAY	Herbal Infusions for Hormonal Balance	Berry and Chia Seed Pudding	Detox Salad with Lemon-Tahini Dressing	Zucchini and Chickpea Patties
SATURDAY	Lentil and Vegetable Wrap	Hummus-Stuffed Bell Peppers	Quinoa and Black Bean Soup	Lentil and Vegetable Stew

PRODUCE:

Spinach (2 bunches)
Bell Peppers (assorted, 6)
Quinoa (1 pack)
Fresh Herbs (assorted, 1 bunch)
Zucchini (3)
Tomato (4)
Sweet Potato (2)
Cherry Tomatoes (1 pack)
Red Onion (2)
Cucumber (2)
Kale (1 bunch)
Lemon (2)
Lime (2)
Strawberries (1 pack)
Fresh Cilantro (1 bunch)
Fresh Mint (1 bunch)
Garlic (1 pack)

PROTEINS:

Chickpeas (2 cans)
Lentils (1 pack)
Tofu (1 pack)

GRAINS:

Whole Wheat Wraps (1 pack)

DAIRY AND ALTERNATIVES:

Feta Cheese (1 pack)
Coconut Milk (2 cans)
Almond Butter (1 jar)

BAKERY:

Whole-Grain Bread (1 loaf)

NUTS AND SEEDS:

Almonds (1 pack)
Chia Seeds (1 pack)
Pumpkin Seeds (1 pack)
Sunflower Seeds (1 pack)

PANTRY STAPLES:

Olive Oil
Coconut Oil
Cumin
Cinnamon
Nutmeg
Red Curry Paste
Vegetable Broth (2 cartons)
Diced Tomatoes (2 cans)
Spaghetti (1 pack)
Tahini (1 jar)
Maple Syrup (1 bottle)
Black Beans (2 cans)
Quinoa and Black Bean Salad Ingredients
Brown Lentils
Smoked Paprika
Balsamic Vinaigrette Dressing
Lentil Bolognese Ingredients
Hummus (1 container)
Lemon-Tahini Dressing Ingredients

BEVERAGES:

Herbal Infusions (assorted, 1 box)

	BREAKFAST	SNACK	LUNCH	DINNER
SUNDAY	Quinoa and Black Bean Salad	Almond Energy Bites	Sweet Potato and Chickpea Buddha Bowl	Vegan Stuffed Bell Peppers
MONDAY	Green Smoothie Bowl	Herbal Infusions for Hormonal Balance	Stuffed Bell Peppers with Quinoa	Lentil and Vegetable Stew
TUESDAY	Herbal Infusions for Hormonal Balance	Chocolate Avocado Mousse	Quinoa and Berry Parfait	Plant-Based Stir-Fry
WEDNEDAY	Avocado Toast Variations	Banana-Oat Cookies	Detox Salad with Lemon-Tahini Dressing	Zucchini and Chickpea Patties
THURSDAY	Sweet Potato and Kale Bowl	Guacamole and Veggie Sticks	Mediterranean Chickpea Salad	Spaghetti with Lentil Bolognese
FRIDAY	Chickpea and Spinach Salad	Berry and Chia Seed Pudding	Quinoa and Black Bean Soup	Zucchini Noodles with Tomato Sauce
SATURDAY	Lentil and Vegetable Wrap	Minestrone Soup	Chickpea and Spinach Curry	Lentil and Vegetable Stew

PRODUCE:

Spinach (2 bunches)

Bell Peppers (assorted, 6)

Quinoa (1 pack)

Fresh Herbs (assorted, 1 bunch)

Zucchini (3)

Tomato (4)

Sweet Potato (2)

Cherry Tomatoes (1 pack)

Red Onion (2)

Cucumber (2)

Kale (1 bunch)

Lemon (2)

Lime (2)

Strawberries (1 pack)

Fresh Cilantro (1 bunch)

Fresh Mint (1 bunch)

Garlic (1 pack)

PROTEINS:

Chickpeas (2 cans)

Lentils (1 pack)

Tofu (1 pack)

GRAINS:

Whole Wheat Wraps (1 pack)

DAIRY AND ALTERNATIVES:

Feta Cheese (1 pack)

Coconut Milk (2 cans)

Almond Butter (1 jar)

BAKERY:

Whole-Grain Bread (1 loaf)

NUTS AND SEEDS:

Almonds (1 pack)

Chia Seeds (1 pack)

Pumpkin Seeds (1 pack)

Sunflower Seeds (1 pack)

PANTRY STAPLES:

Olive Oil

Coconut Oil

Cumin

Cinnamon

Nutmeg

Red Curry Paste

Vegetable Broth (2 cartons)

Diced Tomatoes (2 cans)

Spaghetti (1 pack)

Tahini (1 jar)

Maple Syrup (1 bottle)

Black Beans (2 cans)

Quinoa and Black Bean Salad Ingredients

Brown Lentils

Smoked Paprika

Balsamic Vinaigrette Dressing

Lentil Bolognese Ingredients

Hummus (1 container)

Lemon-Tahini Dressing Ingredients

BEVERAGES:

Herbal Infusions (assorted, 1 box)

	BREAKFAST	SNACK	LUNCH	DINNER
SUNDAY	Sweet Potato and Kale Bowl	Banana-Oat Cookies	Chickpea and Spinach Curry	Lentil and Vegetable Wrap
MONDAY	Herbal Infusions for Hormonal Balance	Detoxifying Cucumber Gazpacho	Mediterranean Chickpea Salad	Quinoa and Black Bean Soup
TUESDAY	Green Smoothie Bowl	Guacamole and Veggie Sticks	Stuffed Portobello Mushrooms	Zucchini Noodles with Tomato Sauce
WEDNEDAY	Avocado Toast Variations	Almond Energy Bites	Quinoa and Berry Parfait	Vegan Stuffed Bell Peppers
THURSDAY	Lentil and Vegetable Wrap	Chocolate Avocado Mousse	Quinoa and Black Bean Salad	Plant-Based Stir-Fry
FRIDAY	Chickpea and Spinach Salad	Berry and Chia Seed Pudding	Detox Salad with Lemon-Tahini Dressing	Zucchini and Chickpea Patties
SATURDAY	Quinoa and Black Bean Soup	Hummus-Stuffed Bell Peppers	Sweet Potato and Chickpea Buddha Bowl	Lentil and Vegetable Stew

PRODUCE:

Spinach (2 bunches)
Bell Peppers (assorted, 6)
Quinoa (1 pack)
Fresh Herbs (assorted, 1 bunch)
Zucchini (3)
Tomato (4)
Sweet Potato (2)
Cherry Tomatoes (1 pack)
Red Onion (2)
Cucumber (2)
Kale (1 bunch)
Lemon (2)
Lime (2)
Strawberries (1 pack)
Fresh Cilantro (1 bunch)
Fresh Mint (1 bunch)
Garlic (1 pack)

PROTEINS:

Chickpeas (2 cans)
Lentils (1 pack)
Tofu (1 pack)

GRAINS:

Whole Wheat Wraps (1 pack)

DAIRY AND ALTERNATIVES:

Feta Cheese (1 pack)
Coconut Milk (2 cans)
Almond Butter (1 jar)

BAKERY:

Whole-Grain Bread (1 loaf)

NUTS AND SEEDS:

Almonds (1 pack)
Chia Seeds (1 pack)
Pumpkin Seeds (1 pack)
Sunflower Seeds (1 pack)

PANTRY STAPLES:

Olive Oil
Coconut Oil
Cumin
Cinnamon
Nutmeg
Red Curry Paste
Vegetable Broth (2 cartons)
Diced Tomatoes (2 cans)
Spaghetti (1 pack)
Tahini (1 jar)
Maple Syrup (1 bottle)
Black Beans (2 cans)
Quinoa and Black Bean Salad Ingredients
Brown Lentils
Smoked Paprika
Balsamic Vinaigrette Dressing
Lentil Bolognese Ingredients
Hummus (1 container)
Lemon-Tahini Dressing Ingredients

BEVERAGES:

Herbal Infusions (assorted, 1 box)

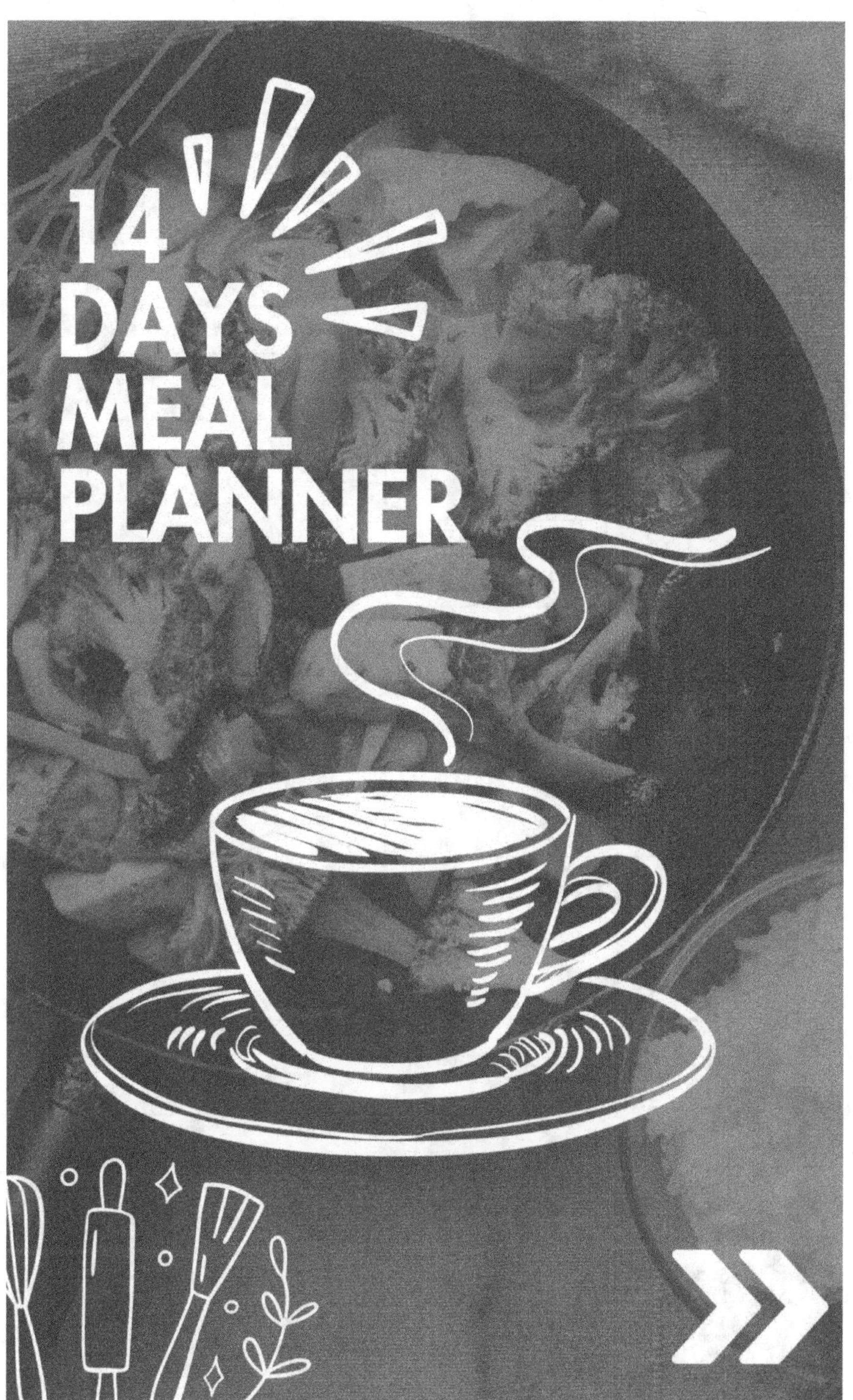
14
DAYS
MEAL
PLANNER

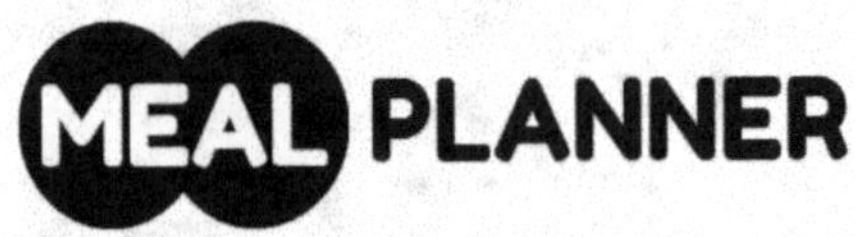
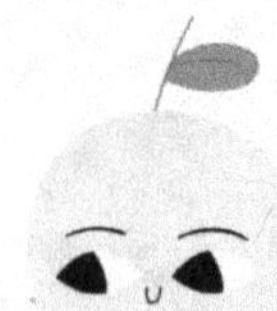

DAY/DATE: _______________________

BREAKFAST

GROCERY LIST

LUNCH

DINNER

SNACKS

NOTES

MEAL PLANNER

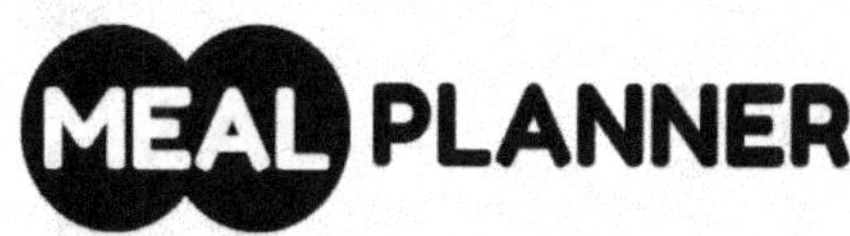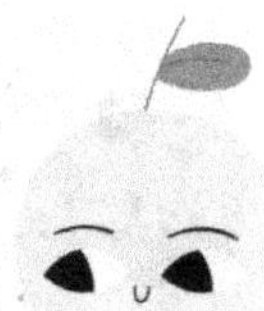

DAY/DATE: _______________________________

BREAKFAST

GROCERY LIST

LUNCH

DINNER

SNACKS

NOTES

DAY/DATE: _______________________

BREAKFAST

GROCERY LIST

LUNCH

DINNER

SNACKS

NOTES

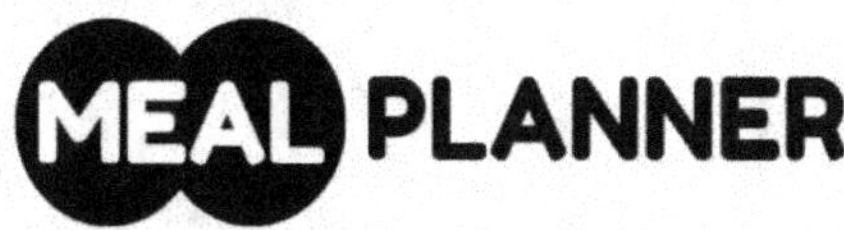 MEAL PLANNER

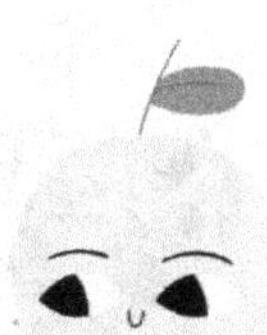

DAY/DATE: _______________________________

BREAKFAST

GROCERY LIST

LUNCH

DINNER

SNACKS

NOTES

MEAL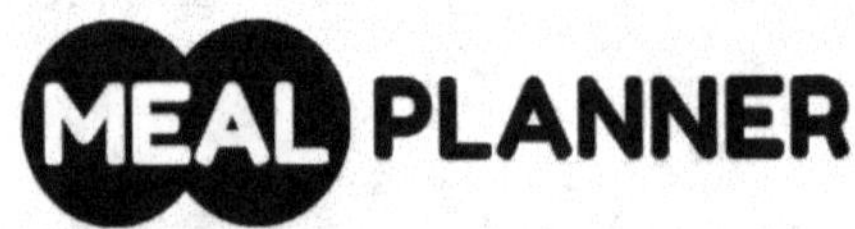 PLANNER

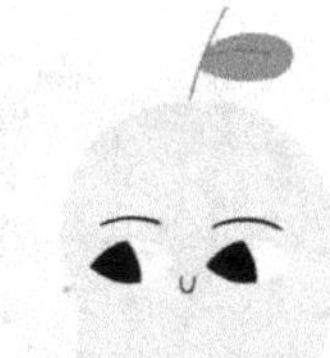

DAY/DATE: _______________________

BREAKFAST

GROCERY LIST

LUNCH

DINNER

SNACKS

NOTES

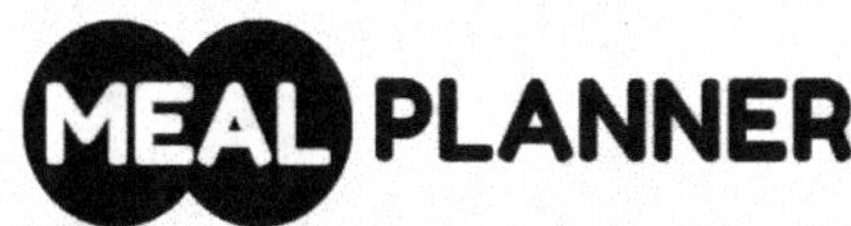

DAY/DATE: _______________________

BREAKFAST

GROCERY LIST

LUNCH

DINNER

SNACKS

NOTES

MEAL PLANNER

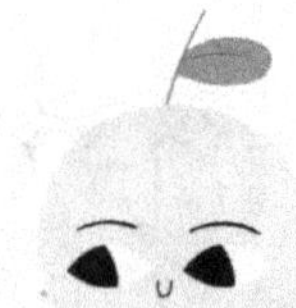

DAY/DATE: ________________________________

BREAKFAST

GROCERY LIST

LUNCH

DINNER

SNACKS

NOTES

MEAL PLANNER

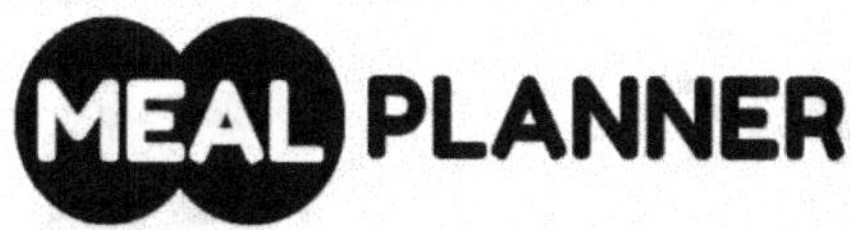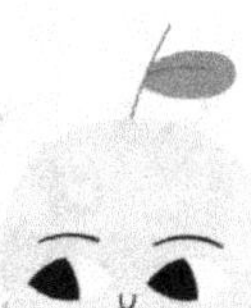

DAY/DATE: ___________________________

BREAKFAST

GROCERY LIST

LUNCH

DINNER

SNACKS

NOTES

MEAL PLANNER

DAY/DATE: _______________________________

BREAKFAST	GROCERY LIST

LUNCH

DINNER

SNACKS

NOTES

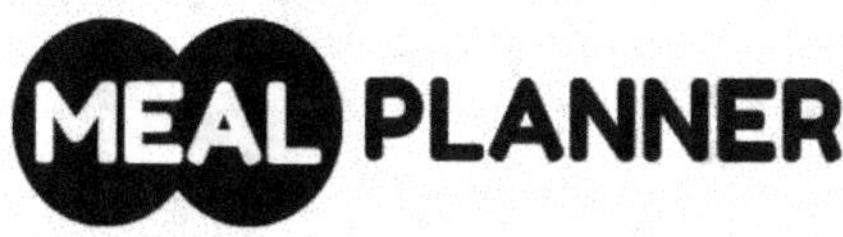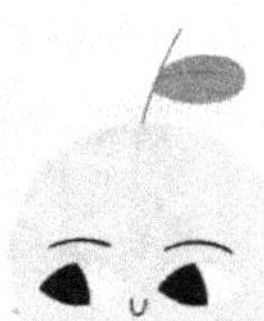

MEAL PLANNER

DAY/DATE: _______________________________

BREAKFAST

GROCERY LIST

LUNCH

DINNER

SNACKS

NOTES

____

____

____

MEAL PLANNER

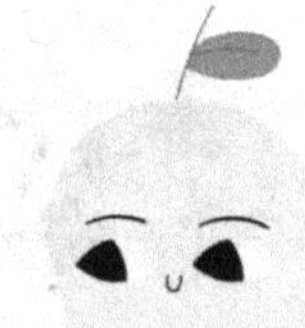

DAY/DATE: _______________________

BREAKFAST

GROCERY LIST

LUNCH

DINNER

SNACKS

NOTES

MEAL PLANNER

DAY/DATE: ______________________

BREAKFAST

GROCERY LIST

LUNCH

DINNER

SNACKS

NOTES

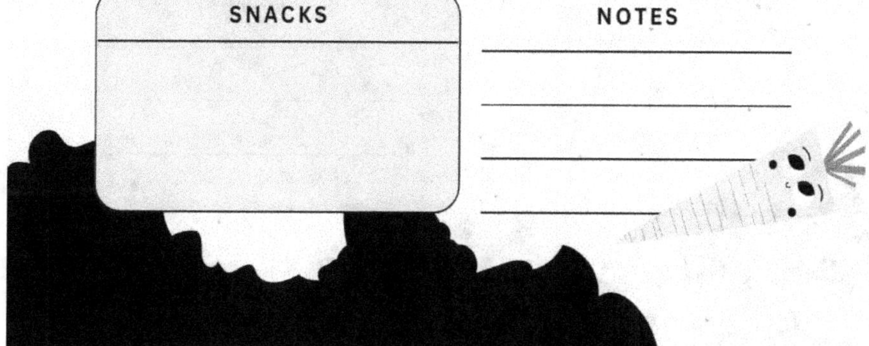

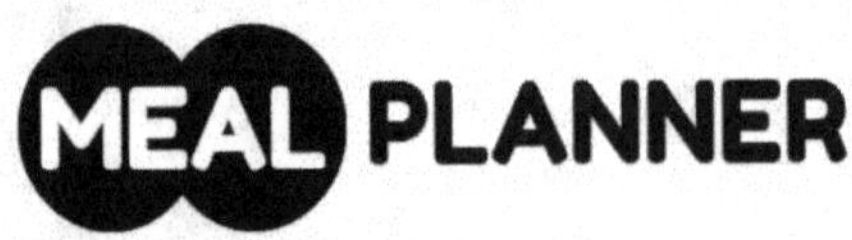 MEAL PLANNER

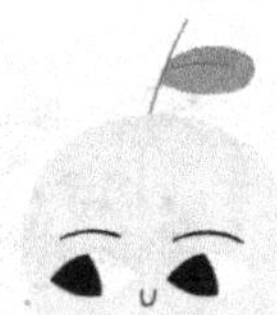

DAY/DATE: _______________________

BREAKFAST

GROCERY LIST

LUNCH

DINNER

SNACKS

NOTES

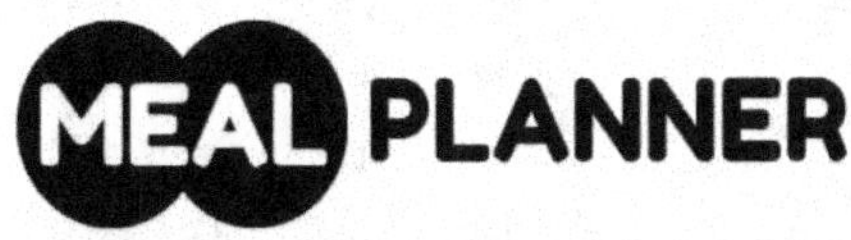 MEAL PLANNER

DAY/DATE: ___________________________

BREAKFAST

GROCERY LIST

LUNCH

DINNER

SNACKS

NOTES

____

____

____

____

- Dash or pinch = >1/8 tsp
- 1-1/2 tsp = 1/2 Tbsp
- 3 tsp = 1 Tbsp; 1/2 fl oz
- 4-1/2 tsp = 1-1/2 Tbsp
- 2 Tbsp = 1/8 C; 1 fl oz
- 4 Tbsp = 1/4 C; 2 fl oz
- 8 Tbsp = 1/2 C; 4 fl oz
- 12 Tbsp = 3/4 C; 6 fl oz
- 16 Tbsp = 1 C; 8 fl oz.; 1/2 pt.

CUP MEASUREMENTS:

- 1/8 C = 2 Tbsp; 1 fl oz
- 1/4 C = 4 Tbsp; 2 fl oz
- 1/3 C = 5 Tbsp + 1 tsp
- 1/2 C = 8 Tbsp; 4 fl oz
- 2/3 C = 10 Tbsp + 2 tsp
- 3/4 C = 12 Tbsp; 6 fl oz
- 7/8 C = 3/4 C + 2 Tbsp
- 1 C = 16 Tbsp; 8 fl oz; 1/2 pt
- 2 C = 1 pt; 16 fl oz
- 4 C = 2 pt; 1 qt; 32 fl oz

PINTS, QUARTS, GALLONS & POUNDS

- 1/2 pt = 1 C; 8 fl oz
- 1 pt = 2 C; 16 fl oz
- 1 qt = 4 C; 32 fl oz
- 1 gal = 4 qt; 16 C
- 1/4 lbs = 4 oz
- 1/2 lbs = 8 oz
- 3/4 lbs = 12 oz
- 1 lbs = 16 oz

METRIC VOLUME:

- 1 ml = 1/5 tsp
- 5 ml = 1 tsp
- 15 ml = 1 Tbsp
- 60 ml = 1/4 C; 2 fl oz
- 80 ml = 1/3 C
- 125 ml = 1/2 C; 4 fl oz
- 160 ml = 2/3 C
- 180 ml = 3/4 C; 6 fl oz
- 250 ml = 1 C; 8 fl oz
- 375 ml = 1-1/2 C; 12 fl oz
- 500 ml = 2 C; 16 fl oz; 1 pt
- 700 ml = 3 C
- 950 ml = 4 C; 32 fl oz; 1 qt
- 1 L = 33.8 fl oz
- 3.8 L = 4 qt; 1 ga

METRIC WEIGHT:

- 1 gr = 0.035 oz
- 100 gr = 3.5 oz
- 500 gr = 17.6 oz; 1.1 lbs
- 1 kg = 35 oz; 2.2 lbs

COOKING TEMPERATURE:

- 0°C = 32°F
- 100°C = 212°F
- 120°C = 250°F
- 160°C = 320°F
- 180°C = 350°F
- 190°C = 375°F
- 205°C = 400°F
- 220°C = 425°F
- 230°C = 450°

www.ingramcontent.com/pod-product-compliance
Lightning Source LLC
Chambersburg PA
CBHW070903260726
48661CB00004B/1569